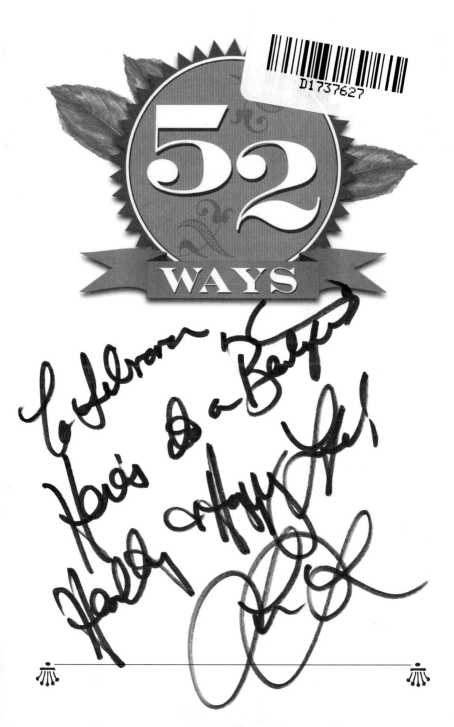

52

WAYS

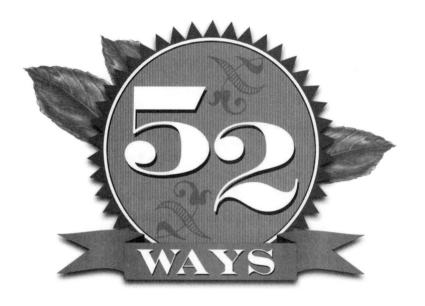

To a Healthy You

Laura Lewis

52 WAYS TO A HEALTHY YOU

Manufactured in the United States of America

For information, please contact:
Brown Books Publishing Group
16200 North Dallas Parkway, Suite 170
Dallas, Texas 75248
www.brownbooks.com
972-381-0009
A New Era in Publishing™

ISBN-13: 978-1-933285-86-3
ISBN-10: 1-933285-86-9
LCCN 2007925304
1 2 3 4 5 6 7 8 9 10

Dedication

To Tarah, Victoria, and Baron

Table of Contents

Foreword

Reading *52 Ways to a Healthy You* was indeed revelational. As a neurologist and psychiatrist, I have been interviewed several times by Laura Lewis in my area of expertise: smell and taste disorders. She is an enlightened interviewer, but she has proven herself beyond the nuncupative in this book. Abundant and useful information is provided here, not just in the areas of smell and taste but also in areas involving essential life situations. I am particularly impressed by her insightful suggestions for approaches in alternative complementary medicine. This book is a must read, not only for the general public but for physicians as well. Laura provides great insight by interpreting relatively dry medical research and applying all to our everyday lives. She has shown herself to be a pioneer in applied medical science and putting it in layman's terms.

I encourage you to go to chapter 20 and review the Holmes-Rahe scale. These life change units have been shown to be predictive of risks of illness. I believe that she so well describes what is routinely ignored by physicians. Her suggestions for managing these changes are easy to follow. As Laura suggests, whatever you learn in this book should be shared with your personal physician to help in your care.

·

My hat is off to Laura for such an outstanding work and I encourage the reader to enjoy and savor this book.

Alan R. Hirsch, MD
Neurological Director, Smell & Taste Treatment and Research Foundation
Chicago IL
Author of *What's Your Food Sign*
www.smellandtaste.org

Preface

Welcome and Congratulations! You have just taken the first step toward taking control of your destiny by beginning this book. Did you know that it is estimated that almost 70 percent of all diseases are a direct result of our lifestyle choices? What you eat and drink, knowing how much stress you are under and how you cope, and your level of physical activity are all part of your lifestyle. If you make incorrect choices now and come from a family with a history of problems such as obesity, diabetes, heart disease, or cancer, your chances of perpetuating the same patterns are extremely high.

I feel certain, however, if you implement some or most of *52 Ways* into your life, you will not only feel and look better soon, but a few decades from now you'll also fare better than your couch potato cohorts! I hope you enjoy *52 Ways to a Healthy You.* Just consider it one of the many tools for acquiring a higher quality of life! Read on and best of luck . . . your life is depending upon you!

Laura Lewis, Dallas, Texas, 2007

Acknowledgments

I am amazed at what my journey has been like since I wrote the first version of this book, *52 Ways to Live a Long and Healthy Life*. Ironically, I had dedicated it to my husband, who suddenly and tragically passed away only one year after its release. Since then, I have had the support of many on my path to recovery from losing one so dear to my heart. On my path to becoming whole again, there were many angels along the way. Barbara Graham, my friend, who helped lead me through the darkness and back into the light of day. Thank you. I thank my girls, Tarah and Victoria, who have become beautiful, vivacious, and intelligent young women with strong and open hearts to the idea that life can be wonderful, in spite of the unpleasant surprises life may bring. Thank you Tarah and Vic for putting up with your mommy's intense desire to make a difference, for supporting me in my writing, and most of all for continuing to believe in dreams. And thank you Baron for those hugs!

Thank you to my mother and father for just being there for me. To Beata, my deepest gratitude to you for all those times you were truly there for us. And of course my sister, Julie, my best friend; thank you.

I would also like to extend sincere gratitude to Tom Colvin and his partners for helping make this book become a reality. My manager, Lyle Walker, you are simply the best. Deb Durham of the Spokesperson's Network, you are fantastic and thank you! To the team at Carry On Media and Pharmavite® for choosing me to lead their campaign with NatureMade® vitamins, thank you!

I want to acknowledge Robbie Durand for his great skill and passion for health research and for providing me with relevant scientific data and friendship during the course of this book's rebirth! Thank you Andrea Gillim for your angelic typing and showing up exactly when I needed you most!

I want to acknowledge the wonderful team at Brown Books: Kathryn Grant for your patience, kindness, and supreme editing skills; Ted Ruybal for the creation of the book cover and layout; and of course, Milli Brown, who is a true mentor to me. Thank you for your belief, creativity, and hard work as partners in this endeavor!

And most of all, I want to thank you dear reader, for giving this book a try. It is my hope you will be motivated to live an extraordinary life.

Introduction

Once you commit to something, life moves in ways you could never have imagined.

—Goethe—

Did You Know: Fifty million Americans suffer from high blood pressure, fifteen million are chronic alcoholics, forty million will spend some time in the hospital each year, sixteen million suffer from ulcers, and over two hundred million are constipated! We have the most modern health care system in the world and still have some of the sickest, fattest, and most malnourished people on earth. What is wrong with this picture? This book provides you with a wide variety of current research and health information and how you can apply it to real life. Your real life!

Your Approach: Skim the table of contents and see the overall picture. *52 Ways . . .* allows you to approach this book on a weekly basis if you so desire. At the end of the year, your health transformation will be complete! Or perhaps you would like to try several of the ways during a one-week time period. If you're of the health elite, you may want to read the entire book over a period of several days, pick up on the items where you feel you need improvement, and act on them. This book also provides food for thought in the form of quotes, Action Tips, and FMI (For More Information).

A Program: It's a progressive health program in disguise! You'll gradually change your diet, become more active and learn how to relax! You'll lose body fat, improve your cardiovascular health and nutritional status, lessen your risk of cancer, and you may even look younger when you've actually completed implementing each action tip.

The Desire to Change: Let's face it. Change can be uncomfortable, especially if you are adopting a new way of being! I encourage you to disregard naysayers and your own negative self-talk. Instead, focus upon each new idea and integrate it into what will become the "new you" . . . or rather the "real you" who deserves to live a happy and joyous life. It is important you believe you deserve nothing but the very best. Taking care of yourself now really will have an impact upon your entire life. If you feel happy, alive, energetic you can change your life for the better in every way. And, best of all, you get to spread the word—at work, at family functions, at parties. Your transformation could become so obvious people will stop you on the street to ask you what you've done. Simply say, "I did it with 52 Ways . . ."

Action Tip:

Ready . . . Set . . . Go! Today is the first day of the rest of your life!

A cheesy profit? Every day, Americans eat
seventy-five acres of pizza!

Do It Right
with Dynamic D

Some pursue happiness...others create it.
—Anonymous—

Did You Know: They say, "The best things in life are free." This may especially be true for vitamin D, which is the only vitamin your body can synthesize directly from sunshine. For years, it was known that D played an important role in the development of strong bones. Recent studies now show vitamin D is important for the maintenance of healthy tissues and has a role in the prevention of certain cancers. Vitamin D has also been discovered to assist in the prevention and treatment of diabetes, certain autoimmune diseases, and cardiovascular disease. D can be produced in the body through the skin's interaction with ultraviolet B radiation, from sunshine or artificial sunlight sources. Once it is produced, it is converted in the body to its active, usable pre-hormone form, called 1,25-dihydroxyvitamin D3.

D History: Vitamin D has an interesting history. As the Industrial Revolution took hold in Europe and the population began to move to growing, smoggy cities in order to find industrial jobs, a mysterious affliction began to strike the children of factory workers in epidemic proportions. This mysterious disease caused children to have bowlegs and was called rickets. It was characterized by skeletal bones that did not harden but remained soft or cartilaginous. In 1822, Polish physician, Jedrzej Sniadecki, noted an odd geographic distribution of rickets cases. Children living in the city were much more likely to develop rickets than those living in the outskirts or in rural areas. He concluded rickets was related to lack of exposure to sunshine. In the 1920s, nutritionists were able to prevent or cure rickets by feeding children cod liver oil. Nutritionists also prevented rickets by exposing children to direct sunlight or light from a sunlamp. The explanation for these findings didn't crystallize for several more years. We now know cod liver oil was effective against rickets because of its high vitamin D content. And, in turn, vitamin D was identified as playing an important role in the hardening of bones.

Functions of Vitamin D: One of vitamin D's most important functions is the regulation of calcium absorption and metabolism. Without sufficient vitamin D, even if there exists sufficient dietary calcium, it will not be properly absorbed and metabolized. Beyond calcium metabolism, vitamin D is now being recognized as critical to a number of other body systems. A deficiency of vitamin D may be associated with many chronic diseases, including common cancers (ovarian, breast, prostate, colon, kidney, and pancreas), autoimmune diseases, such as type 1 diabetes and multiple sclerosis, as well as cardiovascular heart disease, depression, and decreased muscle strength.

The Sun Paradox: It's too bad the news about the exposure to sun and skin cancer relationship has made the public paranoid about getting a little sunshine! It's true, skin cancer is predicted to become an epidemic, and exposure to the sun, is to blame. News reports caution against any unprotected exposure to the sun, and health experts plead with us to stay off the beach and wear either protective clothing or a quality SPF (Sun Protection Factor) lotion. While there is certainly ample evidence that excessive ultraviolet exposure is a risk factor for the development of melanoma (and may cause premature aging of the skin), there is another side to that coin. When our skin is exposed to ultraviolet light, it produces vitamin D. Without sufficient ultraviolet exposure (and a lack of adequate dietary vitamin D to make up for the lost endogenous production), a host of systems in the human body cease to function properly, if at all.

Vitamin D has a powerful inhibitory effect on the growth of many cancers, including, ironically, some skin cancers. While excessive UV light exposure is a known risk factor for the development of melanoma, a chronic vitamin D deficiency created by complete avoidance of unprotected exposure to sunlight will likely lead to a greater risk of developing other cancers or life-shortening disease.

A Key to Preventing the Winter Flu? Every winter, people line up at their doctors' offices to get the flu vaccine, not realizing that vitamin D supplementation boosts the immune system and prevents viral infections. Over the past few years, several researchers have shown that vitamin D significantly enhances antimicrobial peptides and other immune system cells. These antimicrobial proteins help to destroy invading infectious microbes. With their broad-spectrum activity, they are capable of killing everything from bacteria to viruses. Vitamin D—which is produced when the skin is exposed to summer sunlight, and which, conversely, declines in winter—plays a critical role in our vulnerability to influenza infection. Research has shown that macrophages activate vitamin D. The bottom line is that far too many people are deficient in vitamin D, especially the elderly. Unfortunately, by following well-intentioned advice to minimize their exposure to the sun, aging adults may greatly diminish their ability to manufacture optimal levels of vitamin D, particularly compared to young people. This may put them at increased risk of contracting the flu. Most people should supplement with vitamin D especially during the wintertime when there is minimal sun exposure.

"D" Powerful Foods: Few foods contain significant amounts of vitamin D naturally, and the ones that do are foods you don't want to overdo: butter, cream, egg yolks, and liver. Milk is fortified with vitamin D at a level of 100 IU (International Units) per cup. Skim milk is the healthier alternative to whole milk. Some manufacturers fortify cereals with vitamin D. Orange juice is usually vitamin D-fortified. Cod liver oil, as a supplement, contains about 1,200 IU of vitamin D per tablespoon.

D Deficiency: Most people think they get enough vitamin D from sun exposure and dietary sources, such as milk. However, many people actively avoid the sun or use sunscreen to reduce their risk of skin cancer. Aging adults and those with impaired mobility due to chronic disease may become more homebound and not get out in the sun. In the northern United States, available sunshine is not enough to stimulate enough vitamin D formation in the winter. As a result, the prevalence of vitamin D deficiency in the United States has been reported to be as high as 21 to 58 percent in adolescents, 31 percent in adults, and 54 percent in homebound older adults. With only twenty to thirty minutes of sun exposure per day, a fair-skinned person can make a sufficient quantity of vitamin D. A dark-skinned person's body takes about three hours to manufacture an equal amount of the vitamin due to how skin pigments filter out ultraviolet rays.

Vitamin D Supplements: Everyone needs vitamin D. The question is, how much? If your diet lacks vitamin D and/or you are not exposed to the sun's rays, supplementation is necessary for optimal health. In a study of veiled Muslim women in various countries, according to the February 2000 issue of *Journal of Internal Medicine*, it was found the ultimate level of supplemental vitamin D was 1,000 IUs per day. Blood serum levels of 25-hydroxyvitamin D were used to measure vitamin D status. In women who were veiled, who ate a diet low in vitamin D, symptoms of deficiency were evident. In this case, supplementation was necessary and proved to be successful for obtaining and maintaining an optimal healthy state. Most multivitamins offer only the basic level of this nutrient in their formulas. Nature Made Multivitamins with Optimized Nutrient Levels includes 1,000 IUs, the level required for optimal health. The level of vitamin D and other essential nutrients in Nature Made multivitamins are optimized to help repair and strengthen muscle tissue for greater mobility, to support improved heart and organ function, to strengthen the body's ability to protect against the effects of aging, to support mental sharpness, and to maintain cellular health.

FMI:
Nature Made Wellness Advisor Web site: www.NatureMade.com
Nature Made Consumer Affairs Help Line: (800) 276-2878, toll-free

The role of vitamin D in cancer prevention. *Am J Public Health.* 2006
Feburary;96(2):252–61.

·

Estimation of optimal serum concentrations of 25-hydroxyvitamin D for multiple health outcomes. *Am J Clin Nutr.* 2006 Jul;84(1):18-28.

Each square inch of human skin consists of twenty feet of blood vessels.

Bump up Your C!

We should all be concerned about the future because we will have to spend the rest of our lives there.

—Charles F. Kettering—

Did You Know: Longevity seekers, the secret to a long life is right under your nose. You can find it in oranges, berries, cantaloupe, and even in potatoes. It's a vitamin that is one of the supreme leaders of the "the seek and destroy free radicals" club. The major scavenger of cancer-causing cells and one of the best immune system boosters around, ascorbic acid or vitamin C is at the top of the list of life extenders. Eat and ye shall live a long and healthy life! Researchers are finding there really is more to this vitamin C ruckus than just plain old fanaticism and folklore!

C the Basics: Vitamin C is a nutrient that is vital for the proper growth and repair of your tissues, blood vessels, gums, cartilage, and bone. Your skin relies heavily on C because of C's intimate relationship with collagen. Collagen keeps our skin youthful and elastic. Your immune system likes vitamin C because it boosts your body's ability to fight infection. And, good ol' C helps other nutrients enter the bloodstream and be utilized more effectively. According to Dr. Linus Pauling, the Nobel prize-winning proponent of vitamin C, this vitamin may also suppress growth of human leukemia cells; neutralize poisons in your body from pollution, radiation, pesticides; help diabetics have better control of insulin; reduce water retention in tissues; improve male fertility; and prevent heart disease and cancer.

Signs of Low C: If eating fresh fruits and vegetables is not on your list of priorities, a deficiency of Vitamin C is a likely result. Bleeding gums, a tendency to bruise easily, pain or swelling in your joints, nosebleeds, anemia, lowered resistance to infections, and wounds or broken bones that take a longer than usual time to heal could all easily be signs of a lack of vitamin C. The vitamin C Recommended Dietary Intake, or RDI, for the average person under the age of fifty-five is 60 milligrams per day. Pregnant women need 80 milligrams and breast-feeding women need 120 milligrams. Most animals are able to synthesize vitamin C in their bodies. Because human beings can't produce vitamin C, and C is needed for optimal health, we must get it in our diets.

Vitamin C Terminators: We are all biochemically unique, which means not one of us has identical nutritional needs. On a typical day, we use up the vitamin C floating around in our blood streams every two to three hours. Hence, eating a diet that is high in vitamin C is essential for optimal health. There are also a variety of factors that make our C burn up faster. Vitamin C is water-soluble, making it more volatile, so that it is used up quickly and, therefore, doesn't really hang around in your system very long. If you smoke, your vitamin C needs skyrocket because smoking literally burns up the C. Stress also eats up C at a fairly brisk pace.

S'more C facts:

- Several large population studies have shown a reduction in cardiovascular disease in association with vitamin C. For example, a 1992 study that evaluated 11,348 men over a ten-year period reported that men who took 800 milligrams a day of vitamin C lived six years longer than those who consumed the FDA's Recommended Daily Intake (RDI) of 60 milligrams a day. The study concluded that high vitamin C intake extended average life span and reduced mortality from cardiovascular disease by 42 percent.

- When taking vitamin C, it should be consumed in conjunction with vitamin E. Vitamin E has been specifically shown to regenerate vitamin C in the blood. A study reported similar findings in a nine-year study involving 11,178 participants. It showed that people who took vitamin C and E supplements experienced a 42 percent reduction in overall mortality.

- In addition to being a potent antioxidant, vitamin C is also a vasodilator. A vasodilator opens up your blood vessels facilitating more blood flow through your arteries. Impaired vasodilatation is observed in patients with heart failure, high cholesterol levels, hypertension, diabetes, and in smokers. Vasodilatation in patients with heart disease is significantly improved following supplementation with 500 milligrams of vitamin C per day for thirty days and is comparable to vasodilatation seen in healthy people. In addition, another study demonstrated that 500 milligrams of vitamin C per day given for thirty days lowers blood pressure in moderately hypertensive patients. High blood pressure is a major risk factor for heart disease.

- Researchers have found endurance athletes might benefit from adding extra vitamin C to their diets. They found vitamin C supplements, along with vitamin E, reduced tissue damage and sped up post-event recovery.

- In almost 100 percent of cases of women with abnormal pap smears, where cervical dysplasia was diagnosed, there was a vitamin C deficiency. In one study, women with this condition who took a supplement of 1,000 milligrams of vitamin C per day for six months experienced complete recovery from the condition!

- Cataracts that develop in the elderly might be prevented with vitamin C and E supplements. Some researchers believe the cataracts are forming as a result of free radicals floating around. As we age our disease-fighting capabilities drop. Free radicals (the bad guys) are given a chance to do their dirty work if vitamin C levels are low.

- Vitamin C has been found to have a protective effect against cancer of the esophagus, mouth, stomach, pancreas, cervix, rectum, and breast.

- According to a National Center for Health Statistics nationwide survey on a link between vitamin C and mortality, there was a 35 percent lower death rate in men taking vitamin C supplements than expected, and 10 percent fewer deaths among women.

- Semen has eight times more vitamin C than is normally found in the blood stream. Men who don't get enough vitamin C may increase the risk of sperm cell damage, which may increase the risk of birth defects, genetic disease, and cancer of newborn babies.

Action Tips:

- Eat three to five fresh fruits and vegetables per day. Be sure to include at least one high vitamin C source daily.

- Drink orange juice or other juices high in vitamin C with your iron fortified cereal in the morning.

- Eat broccoli, naturally rich in vitamin C, with your red meat. Iron and vitamin C have a healthy synergy, as vitamin C enhances this blood-fortifying mineral's absorption in the body!

- When cooking veggies, do so in a minimal amount of water and bake, grill, or steam when possible.

- Prepare fresh orange or grapefruit juice if possible. Drink your store orange juice within two to three days of opening the carton.

- Cook your potatoes with the skins on!

- Great sources of vitamin C are oranges, strawberries, raspberries, cantaloupe, watermelon, peppers, broccoli, and cauliflower.

- If supplementation seems attractive, try Ester-C®. It's a form of vitamin C with a few metabolites attached to each C molecule, making it work more like a food within your body. Consequently, Ester-C® is absorbed into your bloodstream four times faster than normal vitamin C supplements. Nature Made's Advanced Ester-C® contains phytonutrients and bioflavanoids. Go to the web at www. naturemade.com or look for this product in your local pharmacy or grocery store.

•

FMI:

How to Live Longer and Feel Better and *Vitamin C, the Common Cold and the Flu,* Dr. Linus Pauling, Avon Publishing, New York, 1987

The human body has forty-five miles of nerves.

🙊

Light up Your Life

Whoever is happy will make others happy too.
—Anne Frank—

Did You Know: We existed on this earth for many thousands of years with natural sunlight, fire, and torches as the only means to illuminate our lives. Artificial light sources such as fluorescent and incandescent light bulbs do not provide the same quality of rays as the sun. If one basks in the sun too often, of course, there is a heightened risk of skin cancer and eye problems due to the high level of exposure to ultraviolet (UV) rays. But guess what? A little bit of UV may actually be beneficial to your health!

Rays Your Curiosity: Imagine natural sunlight having the same color qualities as a rainbow. As a matter of fact, a rainbow is an excellent example of what white light or sunlight really looks like under very special conditions. Each color of the rainbow has a different quality in that individual rays are made up of different wavelengths. Natural sunlight is made up of the total combination of a full spectrum of colors. Artificial lighting will vary; some bulbs may contain a lot of blue but perhaps be missing some of the colors found in the rainbow. Other bulbs might be pinker, etc. Radical researchers from this country as well as from Russia have speculated for decades that lack of natural or full spectrum light may be deleterious to our physical and mental health.

A Smidgen of Sunshine: Too much sun leads to skin cancer; however, too little sun may be worse. Sunshine is needed for the production of vitamin D. Vitamin D is nicknamed the "sunshine vitamin" because the skin manufactures it from ultraviolet rays. Getting just the right amount of sun is actually good for your health. Most recently, vitamin D increasingly has been reported to be important for preventing and even treating many types of cancer. This powerful vitamin has been found to protect against lymphoma and cancers of the prostate, lungs, and, ironically, the skin. The strongest evidence is how powerful vitamin D is at protecting against colon cancer. (See "Dynamic D.")

A SAD affair: Seasonal affective disorder, or SAD, is acknowledged in the psychiatric community as a disorder where light deprivation might cause depression or the blues. The northeastern and northwestern states do not have as much annual sunshine as other parts of the country. Depression and suicide rates are higher in cloudy states than in sunshine states such as Florida. Apparently, the way your eye receives light impacts your pituitary gland, which is the master controller of your endocrine or hormonal release system. Because SAD sufferers lack exposure to natural sunshine during cloudy, rainy seasons, medical experts have brought the sunshine inside, via a special light unit that patients use therapeutically in homes or offices! Exposure is limited to short periods of time, keeping in mind that too much sunlight (natural or artificial) can be harmful to health. The light, in some way, impacts the production of "happy" hormones and alleviates the depression if it is indeed light deprivation-related.

Another Eye-Opener: Your sunglasses, which filter out harmful UV rays, might protect your eyes from sun damage due to overexposure. But a little bit of sunlight, including UV rays allowed to directly enter your eyes, might make you feel better! Many regular eyeglasses, contact lenses, and glass windows in cars, homes, and offices filter out the "healthy" rays. These healthy rays, if allowed to enter the pupil of your eye directly (sitting in the shade of a tree on a sunny day will do the trick), appear to impact your immune system favorably. Although scientific studies are limited in this area, many people with arthritis, low energy, low sex drive, etc. improve after purposefully getting a sun fix or replacing regular light bulbs with those that have full-spectrum light.

Light Tidbits: Although other aspects of the benefits of exposure to natural or full spectrum light are not fully scientifically documented, take a look at a few situations that might illuminate the possibilities:

- Mating patterns in many species of birds, reptiles, and animals are directly related to exposure to varying degrees of light and dark, as naturally presented through the seasons! Zookeepers can attest to increased appetites, activity, and fertility in animals when their lighting conditions were improved.

- Bumping up hens' exposure to light, making days last longer, can increase commercial egg production.

- Fertility rates go down in many animal species if exposure to natural sunlight or full-spectrum light is limited completely.

- Blue-light therapy is used to alleviate certain types of jaundice in newborn babies. The natural-type light enhances normal glandular function.

- Psoriasis sufferers benefit from exposure to natural sunlight or limited exposure to black lights (UV).

- When exposed to full-spectrum lighting or more natural sunlight, hyperactive children in classrooms calmed down!

- Productivity in workers increases with full spectrum lighting, citing less fatigue and illness!

- People who wear rose- or pink-tinted glasses may be a little more emotional or irritable than those who wear medium gray lenses. The former director of the Kansas City Royals Baseball Academy said he calmed down an aggressive player by changing his lenses from pink to gray!

- Rats kept in the dark for extended periods of time and given the choice between water and alcohol chose alcohol as the preferred beverage.

Action Tips:

- Make an effort to get a daily sun fix.

- Venture outside for about an hour a day; take off your glasses. Do not look directly at the sun. Sitting in the shade of a tree or umbrella is effective. Even on cloudy days, the rays still come through. To protect your skin, be sure always to wear sunscreen.

- Researchers are not suggesting that you fry on a beach. But many scientists believe that "safe sun"—fifteen minutes or so a few times a week without sunscreen—is not only possible but also healthful.

- Buy full-spectrum bulbs that contain UV. Check out new bulbs designed to fit in regular lamps. Older full spectrums used to be available only in long fluorescent tubes.

- Open windows when weather permits in order to allow some healthy light to enter!

- The sun cheers us. The warm rays on our body give us a psychological boost to our well-being. Our brains produce a chemical called serotonin, which is responsible for controlling our moods. And if you are enjoying yourself you are more likely to laugh, which releases endorphins, the body's natural feel-good chemicals, which can help reduce many diseases.

- If you work nights without full-spectrum lighting, and sleep days, try to get at least an hour of natural light exposure, especially if you feel fatigued, lethargic, and your immune system isn't up to speed

---

FMI:
The National Organization for SAD (NOSAD)
www.nosad.org

Society for Light Treatment and Biological Rhythms (SLTBR)
SLTBR, 4648 Main Street Chincoteague, VA 23336
www.sltbr.org

The Circadian Lighting Association
www.claorg.org

Dr. Norman Rosenthal, MD, coined the term "SAD."
www.normanrosenthal.com

A person will burn approximately two and a half calories by melting an ice cube in his or her mouth.

Create a Little Resistance

Use it or lose it.

—Jimmy Connors—

Did You Know: The easiest way to keep your metabolism revved, improve the health of your heart and lungs, keep your bones strong and healthy, and keep your mind sharp is to include a little resistance in your life! Resistance training is also known as strength or weight training. The importance of aerobic exercise and how it relates to health has been emphasized dramatically over the past two decades with resistance training taking a back seat . . . until the American College of Sports Medicine actually set up guidelines for "balanced fitness." Balanced fitness includes regular aerobic exercise at least three times per week for a minimum of thirty-minute duration, in addition to two resistance-training sessions of moderate intensity per week.

Strength by Definition: According to the National Strength and Conditioning Association (NSCA), "Strength training is the use of progressive resistance methods to increase one's ability to exert or resist force." And as we now know, it provides a wide variety of health benefits.

The Good Ol' Swedes: A study was conducted in Sweden in 1971 that compared the bone strength of professional and world-class athletes, recreational athletes, and nonexercisers. They were divided into groups according to the type of exercises they performed. These exercises included running, swimming, weight lifting, and soccer. The professionals had stronger bones than the recreational and nonexercising groups. The recreational group had stronger bones than the inactive individuals. Who had the strongest bones over all? The weight lifters! The results of the study caught the eye of the scientific community, spawning many more studies to be directed towards resistance exercise and how it will impact one's health.

Structure in Flux: Your bones are not dead material. Old bone cells are constantly dying and new ones are being created. As we get older, especially as we get on up to our senior years, bone loss, or osteoporosis, is common and is mostly due to lessened activity levels. The typical pattern: we get older, a little stiffer, and less mobile. Therefore, less force is placed upon the bones, making them weaker. The results of the Swedish study and many others that followed have concluded that some form of resistance training will make your bones stronger, even if you're in your eighties!

Not Just for Bones: Aerobic exercise is commonly known to lead to improved heart health and function. New research suggests weightlifting alone promotes healthy hearts. Harvard University researchers studied the role different types of exercise play on heart disease risk. Among more than 44,000 men who participated in the Health Professionals Follow-Up Study, those who lifted weights for thirty minutes or more, at least once a week, showed a cardiac risk reduction of 23 percent.

"GET" Those Hormones Revved: We lose muscle mass as we age due to a reduction in circulating hormones that facilitate the building of muscle. Anabolic hormones make our muscles strong and reduce body-fat. The top three hormones that decline dramatically throughout our life cycle are: growth hormone, estrogen, and testosterone or "GET"! The GET hormones skyrocketed when you were in your teens and gave you that youthful feeling. You GET excited, energized, and happy when these hormones are at an all-time high! Our body naturally produces these hormones, yet, for some reason, they diminish as we age. Keeping hormones at a more youthful level is possible. Resistance exercise has been shown to increase the magical GET mix of hormones leading to an increase in your lean muscle. Fat stores are reduced too, regardless of your age.

The "Meat" of the Muscle Story:

- If you don't exercise at all, after the age of twenty you will begin to lose one-half pound of muscle per year. Losing one-half pound of muscle will drop your metabolic rate by .5 percent or 50 calories.

- You have over 600 muscles in your body and over six billion muscle fibers! One muscle fiber can support up to one thousand times its own weight.

- Did you know you have the same number of muscle fibers as you did when you were born? They've just grown in size!

- People who lose weight on a diet, without exercising at all, will, for each pound lost, lose approximately one-quarter of a pound muscle and three-quarters of a pound of fat. Exercisers on balanced diet plans can lose pounds that are 85 percent fat, instead of just 75 percent fat!

- For every pound of muscle we gain, we increase our metabolic rates by 50 calories per day.

- NASA has found astronauts have a tremendous amount of bone loss when subjected to weightlessness for extended periods of time. What has been concluded is that just the sheer act of gravity pulling upon the bones stresses them enough for them to want to rebuild and become stronger.

Benefits, Benefits: Getting involved in some form of resistance-training program twice a week not only can make your muscles and bones stronger but also strengthens tendons and ligaments, improves your self-image, releases natural opiates or endorphins that improve your moods, increases mental acuity, and makes you look and feel better!

- A woman will not get bulked up like a man, simply because men have testosterone, a male hormone, which females do not produce in mass quantities.

- The best physical results have been found when people who were trying to lose body fat and increase their metabolic rate exercised aerobically three to five times per week and incorporated some form of resistance workout, two to three times weekly.

Action Tips:

- Choose the type of resistance exercise that you are most attracted to. You can work out at home in a home gym with free weights or resistance bands while accompanied by a fitness video.

- Seek advice from a trainer who is certified by the ACSM (American College of Sports Medicine), the Cooper Aerobics Clinic in Dallas, The National Strength and Conditioning Association, or ACE (American Council on Exercise).

- Always warm up before a resistance workout, whether you're going to work out with small dumbbells or cans of pinto beans! A proper warm-up includes increasing your body temperature with movement, such as a short spin on a stationary bike, as well as mimicking the motion you will be going through during the actual weight-lifting process.

- Be conscious of your breathing—always breathe in through your nose before you move and out through your mouth on the maximal exertion of a specific movement.

- Don't go overboard. Take it a little at a time in order to allow your body to slowly build strength without causing undo physical stress! If it hurts, don't continue!

- Space your resistance workouts forty-eight hours apart to give adequate time for repair of your muscle tissues to take place.

- Stretch out each muscle group as you complete your various resistance exercises.

- Be sure your doctor says it's okay to begin a resistance program. Some people with high blood pressure are not able to perform strenuous weight-lifting exercises. You should also note that recent studies have found weight lifting to be destructive to the results of eye surgery if performed within the past year.

- Begin a program and stick with it for at least four to six weeks. You will look and feel better if you are on a well-balanced diet, exercising aerobically for thirty to forty-five minutes, three to five times per week, and including resistance workouts two to three times per week.

·

FMI:
Contact The American College of Sports Medicine,
Box 1440, Indianapolis, IN 46206-1440. Phone: 317-637-9200

They have over 20,000 members in the international, national, and regional chapters. The ACSM is a solid source for obtaining educational material regarding exercise in general.

Fifty percent of Americans drop their exercise programs after six months.

Bring on the Broccoli

*Anybody who knows everything should be taught
a thing or two.*
—Franklin P. Jones—

Be Broccoli Bright: Broccoli is a member of the Brassica family of vegetables. Its siblings include Brussels sprouts, cauliflower, collards, kale, mustard, cabbage, rutabaga, and turnips. Although former President George Bush nixed broccoli in the White House, our overall consumption has increased 900 percent. In 1970 the average person only ate one-half pound of broccoli per year. Now the average is up to four and a half pounds.

A Nutritional Gold Mine: Broccoli is loaded with twice the vitamin C of an orange, loads of beta-carotene or pro-vitamin A, and tons of fiber. Scientists have known for years that people who eat vegetables from the Brassica family are less likely to get colon, stomach, breast, and certain other cancers.

Broccoli Babies: The little guys have more power too! The younger sprouts of broccoli provide a more concentrated amount of beneficial phyto-nutrients than the mature plant. Isothiocyanates, potent cancer fighters, are up to 100 percent higher in young broccoli sprouts than in adult broccoli stalks.

The Life Extender: Also known as a cruciferous vegetable, broccoli may contain the most life-extending nutrients. Broccoli is unusually rich in phytochemicals that fight cancer, including indoles, isothiocyanates, and glucoraphanin, which the body converts to sulforaphane. Sulforophane is a member of the Brassica family. These are enzymes that stimulate the manufacture of "good" types of chemicals, which block carcinogens from developing nasty tumors. When sulfuraphane, which gives the pungent taste to broccoli, was isolated in a lab and given to mice in quantities equivalent to three-quarters of a pound, they were 50 percent less likely to develop cancer!

Action Tip: If you want to lower your risk of cancer, loading up on members of the Brassica family of vegetables should be a part of your diet plan. Eat one-half cup daily. Be careful if your intestines are sensitive to fiber. Steam, don't boil. Steaming will retain most of the beneficial qualities in the vegetable. If you want to be really adventurous and have conditioned your intestines to your new friends, dip raw members of this family into salsa and munch away. Organically grown vegetables are better, but don't forget to wash the little tykes thoroughly.

One in three Americans always feel rushed.

Laugh It Off

Everything is funny as long as it is happening to somebody else!

—Will Rogers—

Did You Know: Laughing one hundred times during a twenty-four hour period has the same cardiovascular benefit as rowing a rowing machine for ten minutes! So says the king of laughter researchers—psychiatrist, William Fry. The reason laughing is so beneficial to your health is because during the actual act of chortling your blood pressure and heart rate rise. Then, after laughter is ceased, your blood pressure and heart rate drop a little lower than where they started. A cardiovascular benefit is the result. Dr. Fry is not saying this will replace your daily walk or trip to the gym or aerobics class. He is saying you need to laugh a little bit more. The most exciting thing about the laughter/health benefit phenomenon is that you can fake a laugh and still receive the same benefits!

Go On and Laugh! According to Mr. Webster's handy pocket dictionary, a laugh is "an expression of mirth or joy by an explosive noise." When this "explosive expression" occurs, your blood flow actually speeds up, reacting to hormones released; and your cancer-fighting ability increases because more of those T-cells can be found floating around your bloodstream, boosting your immune system. Your perception of pain is decreased and the amount of stress-inducing hormones is lowered in your blood stream, making you less stressed! In a laugh study of five men who viewed a sixty-minute videotape of a comedian, measurements of the very hormones that cause stress were taken. The laughing men's blood levels were measured before, during, and after their humorous experience. Levels of epinephrine, cortisol, and dopamine were measured because they are typically high when one is under stress. The result? All levels were lower than before the session.

Laughing Makes a Heart Happy: Laughter lowers blood pressure and heart disease. People who laugh heartily on a regular basis have lower standing blood pressure than the average person. When people have a good laugh, initially their blood pressure increases, but then it decreases to levels below normal. Breathing then becomes deeper which sends oxygen enriched blood and nutrients throughout the body. Laughter may also protect the heart. Laughter, along with an active sense of humor, may help protect you against a heart attack, according to a study at the University of Maryland Medical Center. Researchers found laughter may help prevent heart disease. They also concluded that those individuals who had already developed heart disease were 40 percent less likely to laugh in a variety of situations compared to people of the same age who had healthy cardiovascular systems.

A Smile Is Your Umbrella: It turns out that simply smiling, even if you're not really happy, can also have a positive physical and psychological impact. A negative effect also occurs if you frown or have a look of fear upon your face. Paul Ekman, of the University of California at San Francisco, found that if a person mimics an emotion, his body will respond as if the emotion is really being experienced. If you smile, your body will think you're happy and respond accordingly. Robert Zajonc of the University of Michigan says when we smile we contract forty-two facial muscles. This constriction slows down the blood flow to the brain, via your sinuses, resulting in cooler blood reaching the hypothalamus located within the brain. Your hypothalamus is the master controller of body temperature and emotion. It appears that if cooler blood reaches "the controller," you will experience more pleasant feelings. On the other hand, if the blood is heated up internally (which has nothing to do with the temperature in your environment), you will probably be more stressed out and a little more "hot headed." And one study of students at the University of Illinois who, thinking they were being tested for psychomotor function, were told to clench pens in their teeth, which revealed that when they were mimicking a smiling clench they felt happier!

Action Tips:

- Smile more—when engaged in conversation, driving in your car, even working at the office. Keep in mind the healthy benefits of a smile.

- Do things that make you laugh. Be around people who are "up," and share the fun in life!

- Listen to music that makes you happy!

- Be conscious of your facial expressions. If you look sad and you have no reason to be, try to look happier.

- Chuckle, chortle, giggle, snicker whenever you can, but use discretion so that your friends, boss, or spouse won't think you've gone off the deep end! Or, better yet, let them in on your secret so they can feel better, too.

FMI:
"The Far Side" by Gary Larson

The average woman's thighs are one and a half inches larger in circumference than the average man's.

Make Picasso Proud

*Tell me what you eat
and I will tell you who you are.*

—Anthelme Brillat-Savarin—

Did You Know: Varying the types of food you eat, in accordance with their color, texture, and flavors from meal to meal and day to day, will contribute to a healthier body and mind. One of the tricks to obtaining optimal nutrition from the food you eat is literally to become an artist with your plate!

Your Plate Is Your Canvas: View your plate as an artist's round canvas. You need to not only compose a "painting" or "picture" that contains a variety of colors, but also textures. Make your plate look like a rainbow of colorful food choices: add tomatoes, pink grapefruit, cherries, and watermelon for a touch of red; spinach, kale, broccoli, and zucchini for green; carrots, squash, oranges, and cantaloupe for yellow and orange; blueberries, plums, and blackberries for purple and blue; and onions, white beans, garlic, and leeks for white.

The more color that you have on your plate, the richer it will be in vitamins, minerals, and cancer-fighters. Including various textures, such as leafy greens, baked sweet potatoes, steamed red potatoes, brown rice, whole grain pasta, and legumes such as black beans (high in iron!) or pinto beans, will provide a wide variety of high energy carbohydrates, cancer-fighting fiber, and other types of vitamins and minerals. Varying flavors is also a great way to obtain different nutrients—as long as the flavors aren't from artificial flavorings! Fish and chicken are excellent sources of lean protein. However, keep in mind that if you eat a well-balanced diet with plenty of whole grains, which also provide some protein, the amount of animal protein that you need in an entire day doesn't really need to exceed eight ounces.

Let's Play Picasso: Design your plate to look like the following:

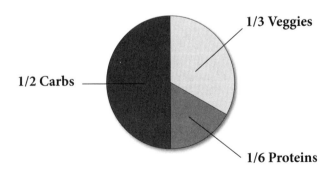

(Plate divided into sections, 1/2 carbs, 1/3 veggies, 1/6 proteins)

Action Tips:

- Always be conscious of creating a "painting" with your food. When you visit a salad bar, be adventuresome and try some bright red beets or shredded carrots or perhaps some sprouts on your salad. Stay away from the carrot salad, potato salad, and anything else with a "fat aura."

- When ordering in a restaurant, try to visualize what your plate will look like. Will it include a great mix of colors and textures? If it doesn't make the grade, order a salad and a side of vegetables or a baked potato sans butter, sour cream, bacon, and cheese! Ask for some salsa to give your potato a great vitamin C and beta-carotene boost!

FMI:
The USDA Food Pyramid
www.mypyramid.gov

---

*The average person ingests approximately one ton
(2,240 pounds) of food and drink per year.*

Get Your ZZZs!

We are all part of the human race, but racing faster will not make me more human.

—Anonymous—

Did You Know: If you have trouble getting to sleep or staying asleep, you're not alone! More than 100 million Americans have occasional sleep problems; one in six is known to have chronic, disruptive insomnia; and more than 80 percent of us are sleep-deprived!

Sleep or Not to Sleep: A short-lived bout of insomnia is generally nothing to worry about. The bigger concern is chronic sleep loss, which can contribute to health problems.

- Learning and memory: Sleep helps the brain commit new information to memory through a process called memory consolidation. In studies, people who had slept after learning a task did better on tests later.

- Metabolism and weight: Chronic sleep deprivation may cause weight gain by affecting the way our bodies process and store carbohydrates and by altering levels of hormones that affect our appetite.

- Safety: Lack of sleep contributes to a greater tendency to fall asleep during the daytime. These lapses may cause falls and mistakes such as medical errors, air traffic mishaps, and road accidents.

- Mood: Sleep loss may result in irritability, impatience, inability to concentrate, and moodiness. Too little sleep can also leave you too tired to do the things you like to do.

- Cardiovascular health: Serious sleep disorders have been linked to hypertension, increased stress hormone levels, and irregular heartbeat.

- Disease: Sleep deprivation alters immune function, including the activity of the body's killer cells. Keeping up with sleep may also help fight cancer.

A Sleepless Society? There are a variety of factors that determine your quality of sleep. Nutritional imbalances; drug interactions; illnesses of your heart, lungs, and digestive systems; hormonal imbalances; pregnancy; and stressful life events such as a death in the family, a wedding, or a demanding new job can all contribute to sleepless nights. The icing on the cake is the anxiety associated with going to bed once

·

you've had a few restless nights. The anxiety by itself will keep you from getting a good night's rest!

When You Sleep: While you are sleeping your body spends most of its energy rebuilding tissues, bones, and many cellular components involved in your circulatory, immune, and hormonal release systems. Most importantly, your brain has time to recover from all of its work. Researchers don't know exactly why, but sleep is essential to your mental health.

How Much Sleep Do We Need? The average adult sleeps seven to seven and a half hours per night. Many people function quite well with only four to six hours sleep. Twenty percent of Americans get less than six hours of sleep per night. Sleep researchers believe the average human being needs not eight but nine hours of sleep in order for the brain to recover from its daily wear and tear.

As a matter of fact, getting an extra hour of sleep, over and above your norm, might give you the equivalent of the energy you receive from two cups of coffee! Researchers have found that if you lose an hour of sleep (for example, if you normally sleep seven hours and you only get six for some reason), your alertness level the next day might be reduced by 20 percent. It could be zombie time after five days of sleep deprivation. Your alertness level could fall by 50 percent. Other researchers have found that most people function quite well following one sleepless night. The sleep-deprived person might feel groggy, but his performance won't really suffer after a one-time deprivation.

Target Your Enemies: Remove any caffeine, alcohol, or nicotine from your daily regimen. Caffeine, especially if drunk six hours or less before bedtime, can disrupt sleep. Alcohol might make you relax enough to fall asleep but often you'll awaken later. Nicotine is a stimulant that could keep you awake as well. Exercising too late in the day might heat up your metabolism and prevent falling asleep easily. Eating too much, too late, or eating spicy foods might also inhibit sleep.

Action Tips:

- Be sure your bedroom is cool.

- Don't use your bedroom for anything but sleeping and sex. Avoid using it as an office or a dining room!

- If you don't fall asleep within fifteen to thirty minutes after lying down, get up and do something relaxing.

- Avoid caffeine, nicotine, and alcohol altogether, and see if you fall asleep more easily.

- Participate in vigorous, aerobic activity in the late afternoon or early evening. Your body's cooling response will enhance sleep.

- Take a calcium-magnesium supplement one hour before bedtime.

- Drink a cup of chamomile tea. It's an herbal tea known for centuries to have a calming effect.

- Avoid using sleeping pills on a regular basis. They do not promote the kind of sleep your brain likes. Try herbal alternatives such as valerian root, which is known to have a similar effect as sleeping pills but is nonaddictive and has no side effects.

- Eat a high carbohydrate dinner and/or snack. This will enhance the release of serotonin, the neurotransmitter that helps you fall asleep!

- Some aromatherapy oils that provide a relaxant effect are chamomile, lavender, neroli, rose, jasmine, sandalwood, Melissa, ylang ylang, and marjoram. Add a few drops to your bathwater or sprinkle a few drops on a handkerchief and inhale.

Dehydration is the major cause of muscle cramps when you are being physically active and is actually a mild form of heat stroke.
—Vitality Magazine

You're "Betta" off
with Beta-carotene

*Never put off until tomorrow what you can do today, because
if you enjoy it today, you can do it again tomorrow.*
—Anonymous—

Did You Know: A sweet potato a day might very well keep
the cancer away! The little tuber is loaded with beta-carotene,
alias pro-vitamin A, which is a precursor to vitamin A. Much
attention has been given to this form of vitamin A and its
carotenoid cousins because of its disease-fighting capabilities. Beta-carotene alone cannot be used by the body. However, when we eat foods high in beta-carotene and digestion
begins, the usable form of vitamin A or retinol is formed as a
result of the breakdown that occurs in the liver and the intestines. Retinol, which is only found in animal foods, does not
appear to have the disease-fighting capabilities that its cousin
beta-carotene has. Studies have shown that individuals who
have eaten diets rich in beta-carotene (and other carotenoids

such as alpha carotene, lutein, lypocene, etc.) over a twenty-year period are less likely to develop certain types of cancer, including lung, mouth, throat, digestive, bladder, skin, and breast cancer. In addition, seniors whose diets are high in beta foods containing carotene are less likely to have cataracts and other problems with their eyes. Recent research studies have shown sweet potatoes to have unique root storage proteins that have significant antioxidant capacities. In one study, these proteins had about one-third the antioxidant activity of glutathione—one of the body's most potent internally produced antioxidants. With higher antioxidants, your body is more likely to fend off disease and maintain optimal health.

What Does It Do For You? Beta-carotene is an antioxidant, which prevents free radicals, or the "bad guys" who cause infection or cancer, from invading your cells. You need vitamin A to keep your skin healthy, to help you to see at night, and to see colors vividly. Vitamin A helps promote growth of all tissues and bone and can prevent respiratory infection by maintaining the health of your mucous membranes.

How Much? There is no set RDA for beta-carotene. If you eat foods daily that contain 6 milligrams (a carrot a day!), you'll meet the RDA equivalent of 5,000 IUs per day. Researchers are experimenting with levels ranging from 15 to 60 milligrams per day, with hopes of finding an optimal level for maximal preventative benefits. Taking a beta-carotene supplement is not necessarily a good thing. A Finnish study of twenty nine thousand smokers actually found an increased risk in lung cancer in men who took beta-carotene supplements. Instead, check out taking a whole-food supplement.

Where Do You Find It? Beta-carotene is found in abundance in orange, yellow and dark green leafy vegetables. Butternut squash weighs in at a hefty thirteen thousand IUs per one-cup serving. Pumpkin and carrots are also high contenders. Sweet potatoes, kale, spinach, cantaloupe, apricots, peaches, mustard greens, and broccoli all contain significant amounts of our buddy, beta-carotene.

The Beta Is Betta Off: Cooked vegetables offer more beta-carotene than raw ones. Fiber can hinder beta-carotene's availability. Cooking breaks down the fibers, making the pro-vitamin A more available. Blanching or steaming is more than adequate to release the "trapped" beta-carotene.

Action Tip: At each meal or snack, be sure to always include a piece of fresh fruit and/or a serving of fresh vegetables. Choose at least one orange or yellow vegetable every other day. Five to nine servings of fresh fruits and vegetables are recommended per day.

In the early 1900s, only 1 percent of the total deaths in the United States were attributed to cancer. In 1992, one in four or 25 percent of all deaths were cancer-related. Since 1991, the total cancer-related deaths have dropped 1 percent each year.

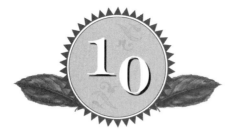

Be "Scentsible"

One should, every day at least, hear a little song, read a good poem, see a fine picture, and, if possible, speak a few reasonable words.

—Johann Wolfgang Von Goethe—

Did You Know: Your sense of smell can directly impact your physical, mental, and emotional state. Despite the tendency of humans to underestimate the role of smell in our everyday lives, for most mammals, it is the most important sense. Dogs are probably the most obvious example of this; it is through the use of smell that animals are able to find food, reproduce, and even communicate. Smell travels directly to the limbic system, one of the oldest parts of the brain. The limbic system is the primitive area of the brain that controls emotions, memory, and behavior. Smell can influence mood, memory, emotions, choice of mate, the immune system, and the endocrine system (hormones). People, for thousands of years, have taken advantage of such a connection by using oils from the seeds, flowers, leaves, bark, and roots of plants to obtain a desired effect. It appears certain fragrances may make you feel calmer, while another may stimulate your senses! These aromas can be used in the form of incense, perfumes, or colognes. The use of these fragrances is called aromatherapy.

Speaking of Experience: The ancient Egyptians were known to have used essential oils, not only in their religious rituals in the form of incense, but Cleopatra was also rumored to use the oil of jasmine as a perfume—apparently Mark Anthony found it rather engaging! Queen Elizabeth II of Hungary, at the wise age of seventy-two, was known to help her own aches and pains caused by gout and rheumatism with a special "toilet water," which contained rosemary, marjoram, and lavender, all known to have antirheumatoid qualities! Aromatherapy is widely used in the countries of Belgium, Germany, Switzerland, England, and France. The French so wholeheartedly believe in the ancient practice that it is even covered by health insurance!

"I'll Have the Lemon Aroma, Please!" In Japan, a very large architectural and construction firm called Shimizu, conducted a one-month study of thirteen keypunch operators. Their number of errors was counted while at the same time having different essential oil aromas released into their work environment! Astonishingly enough, when they breathed in a lavender scent their errors dropped by 21 percent; jasmine decreased the error rate by 33 percent; and lemon essence brought in a whopping 54 percent decrease in mistakes!

"Scents?" You Asked: How can this benefit you? Know this: vanilla and almond scent may make you relax in a stressful situation. This essence was used at Sloan Kettering Cancer Center in New York in eighty-three patients who were undergoing MRIs. When undergoing an MRI you have to lie very still; 10 percent of people usually freak out and ask to be let out—a costly request, as one MRI is expensive. When the vanilla-almond scent was used, their anxiety levels were reduced by 62 percent.

It's All Limbic: We are affected by smells even when we sleep. In a study from Bowling Green State University in Ohio over one hundred college students were tested while they slept. The students experienced an increase in heart rate and brain wave activity when different scents were introduced. It turns out we are highly sensitive to smells, even if we're not conscious of smelling a scent! Dr. Jan Born, from the University of Lubeck in Germany, found new memories can be consolidated while subjects sleep. He and his team introduced the scent of roses during a memory game to volunteers, while others were not exposed to the smell. Then later, during sleep, the same volunteers who smelled the scent were set up in MRI machines and again introduced to the rose essence. Not only did the rose-exposed volunteers remember 97.2 percent of the memory tasks, as compared to 86 percent accuracy in the no-scent recipients, it was also observed the part of the brain associated with new learning was activated when exposed to the rose smell only during deep-wave sleep.

Dr. Gary Schwarz of the University of Arizona studied sub-liminal scents. He was interested in the connection of all the toxic molecules floating around in our unclean environment (paint fumes, smog, cleaning chemicals, gas emissions from new carpeting, and building materials) and the impact they have upon our nervous system. He believed the connection between our sense of smell and our physical, emotional, and mental health is something to be taken seriously. Olfactory scientist, Dr. Charles Wysocki, from the Monell Chemical Senses Center in Philadelphia, explained that when we smell something, the scent or combination of scents is received by a part of your brain, the limbic system, which is directly involved in regulating body functions as well as controlling our emotions.

Smell Alters Reality: Alan Hirsch, MD, a psychiatrist and neurologist and a nationally recognized smell and taste expert, studied how certain scents alter the perception of one's own or someone else's actual weight. Various scents were introduced to groups of fifty men along with no fragrance exposed to a control group. They found the combination of floral and spice affected the men's guess as to how much a 245-pound woman weighed. The floral and spice group guessed, on average, the woman weighed twelve pounds less than her actual weight. Dr. Hirsch speculates certain fragrances can in fact, slightly alter a person's perception of reality as men see women as weighing less than they really do and women perceive them-selves as thinner. In turn, it is possible a favorite perfume may boost a woman's confidence levels. The multibillion dollar fragrance industry has scientific data backing up what may seem to be a frivolous expense.

The Attraction Factor: What contains a compound that elevates women's moods and gets them in the "ready" for romance and increases their stress hormones? Male sweat! Researchers at the University of California Berkley found that women responded specifically to "AND" or androstadienone, a male hormone abundant in men's sweat. By measuring blood pressure, heart rate, breathing, skin temperature, and fidgeting, as well as asking the women certain questions that indicated mood, it was found that indeed the scent of a man can most certainly elicit a hormonal response in women! They also noted there are many other compounds in human sweat that may boost the attraction factor!

Athletes Do It: Runners and triathletes are beginning to find out that by using certain essences their performances have improved. Certain oils can lessen physical and psychological stress, such as lavender, rose, and vanilla-almond oils.

Choices, Choices: Want to relax, or drop your blood pressure? Spiced apple is a sure bet, as well as vanilla. Lavender, chamomile, geranium, and neroli will also make you cool as a cucumber. Get happy with rose, geranium, ylang ylang, rose, clary sage, sandalwood, jasmine, orange blossom, and lemon grass. Sleep like a baby with vanilla-almond, lavender, chamomile, and neroli.

Action Tips:

- Be sure to always use essential oils mixed with an almond or other vegetable oil base if you are going to apply it directly to your skin.

- Try putting a few drops in a bowl of water and let it evaporate slowly.

- Buy a diffuser. Some are designed to fit on a light bulb!

- Burn aromatherapy candles, which contain the true essential oils.

- For jet lag, rub a few drops of lavender, basil, and tangerine on your temples.

- Place a few drops of eucalyptus or rosemary in your bath water to clear your sinuses!

- Do your research first. Sometimes using too much of an essential oil may have the reverse effect you desire.

FMI:
The Smell & Taste Treatment and Research Foundation
845 North Michigan Avenue, Suite 990W
Chicago, IL. 60611 Phone: 312-938-1047
web: www.scienceofsmell.com

*It takes two thousand pounds of roses to make
one pound of rose oil!*

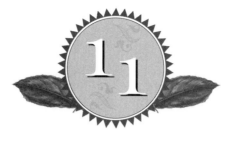

Fiber Your Life

Don't drag the engine, like an ignoramus, but bring wood and water and flame, like an engineer.

—Maria Weston Chapman—

Did You Know: Nine out of ten Americans suffer from clogged colons. Constipation leads to a variety of serious to very serious negative health conditions ranging from varicose veins, hemorrhoids, and high blood pressure to cancers of the colon, stomach, pancreas, breast, and prostate. If things are rather slow in your "interior," you are setting yourself up for a rather unpleasant health scenario in the future. Many negative health problems associated with low fiber begin in childhood and go undetected until they show up in adulthood.

Fabulous Fiber: Fiber is the indigestible part of plant foods. It simply moves through the body without being broken down.

Its purposes are many, but in general, it keeps things moving at the rate they are supposed to. Fiber is actually made up of six different types, which are divided into two groups: soluble and insoluble. Insoluble fiber includes cellulose, hemi-cellulose, and lignin. Insoluble fiber serves to move bulk through your digestive track. It also controls and balances the acidity in your intestines.

Foods that are good sources of insoluble fiber:

- Whole-wheat products

- Wheat oat

- Corn bran

- Flax seed

- Vegetables such as green beans, cauliflowers, and potato skins

- Fruit skins and root vegetable

Soluble fibers are pectin, gums, and mucilages. Soluble fiber binds with cholesterol and inhibits the absorption of cholesterol. It also prolongs stomach-emptying time so that sugar is released and absorbed more slowly into the blood stream.

Soluble fiber can lower total cholesterol and LDL cholesterol (the bad cholesterol); therefore reducing the risk of heart disease by regulating blood sugar.

Some food sources of soluble fiber:

- Oat/Oat bran

- Dried beans and peas

- Nuts

- Barley

- Flax seed

- Fruits such as oranges and apples

- Vegetables such as carrots

- Psyllium husk

A Real Team: Insoluble and soluble fiber work together in order to act as your internal safety guards of your digestive tract. You need about three times the amount of insoluble fiber as you do soluble fiber for optimal health effects. The solubles take up where the insolubles leave off and vice versa.

How Much? The majority of Americans are barely getting one-fifth of the dietary fiber they need. The optimal daily recommendation is 30 to 50 grams. Thousands of years ago, when our ancestors where extremely active, their bodies needed a lot more calories, especially in the form of carbohydrates for energy. Since snack cakes weren't around, fiber rich grains were a primary component of our ancient cousins' diets. Primitive tribes in Africa eat diets close to what our ancient relatives ate. The tribal members have lower cholesterol levels and almost no incidence of hemorrhoids or constipation! In this modern age, we aren't as active as our ancestors, so our calorie needs are lower. But, our digestive tract still wants that large amount of fiber to be healthy!

Fiber "Stars": Many breakfast cereals are great sources of fiber. Kelloggs "Fiber One" and "100% Natural Oat Bran" and "100% Bran" both by Nabisco provide at least 10 grams of fiber in one serving. Apples, blackberries, pears, and strawberries are rich in soluble fiber.

Action Tips:

- Eat at least one-half cup of legumes every other day, if not every day.

- Eat whole grains at every "starch" opportunity, i.e. purchase 100 percent whole grain breads and long-cooking brown rice instead of the white, refined versions.

- Eat a piece of fruit, preferably with the skin at least three times per day.

- Eat plenty of fresh vegetables throughout the day, ordering a side salad to go along with your lunch and dinner. (Avoid saturated fat salad dressings)

- Only eat refined carbohydrates as a "weekly" treat, not on a daily basis.

- Most important of all, if your diet is low in fiber, begin making changes gradually or your digestive tract will rebel! Change to whole grain breads one week. Add beans the next. Add more fruit the next, etc.

Eight-six percent of American children cannot pass a minimum physical fitness test. Only 41.4 percent couldn't pass it in 1954.

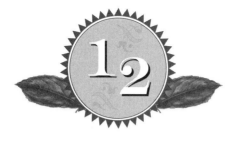

Stretch It Out

If anything is sacred the human body is sacred.
—Walt Whitman—

Did You Know: Stretching your muscles increases the length of your muscle fibers, increases mobility and strength of your joints and spine, and increases blood flow and oxygen to your internal organs and tissues, which in turn increases your energy level. What this means in real life is if you maintain flexibility you'll be able to perform everyday activities without straining tight muscles. If you do not stay active and include a few simple stretches in your everyday routine, you will be stiffer and probably complain about "my aching back" a little more often than your more mobile buddies. If you have ever seen a cat or a dog awaken from a peaceful slumber, you'll often see them stretch their entire body, then amble upon their way. Infants will often stretch upon rising. Stretching is a natural way to keep your muscles and joints flexible.

Stretch Your Limits: You won't find typical Japanese elders sitting in front of Starbucks sipping coffee at 6:00 a.m. You will, however, find them in the park performing Tai Chi. Tai Chi, a form of stretching and breathing exercises, enhances balance and body awareness through slow, graceful, and precise body movements. In the *Journal of the American Geriatrics Society,* it was noted that this ancient healthy practice may significantly cut the risk of falls among older people and help maintain strong and flexible bodies of those who were seventy years of age and older.

A Typical Day: The alarm clock goes off and you jump out of bed to turn it off. A nice, relaxed body contracts and moves suddenly. One of these days you might have a mysterious neck or back strain and not know what caused it. That good old alarm clock will do it every time! You shower, dry off, and begin to dress. You drop your sock on the floor and you bend to pick it up. Ouch! You finish dressing and after coffee you notice your shoe is untied. Can you bend to tie your shoe easily, or are your feeling your age? Driving to work, you find it difficult to look behind you by turning your head. While sitting at your desk at work someone behind you calls your name. Can you turn to look at who's speaking to you without turning your entire body around? If you do not maintain your flexibility, problems may occur with your mobility.

Benefits, Benefits: Regular stretching is physically beneficial in a wide variety of ways besides maintaining mobility.

Stretching:

- Helps keep your spine flexible.

- Decreases natural compression of joints.

- Improves strength.

- Increases circulation to all internal organs and tissues, enhancing their proper functioning.

- Supplies more energy to the body.

- Helps keep bones healthy and strong due to slight pulling on muscles and ligaments that are connected to bones.

- Might relieve constipation by opening the joints and muscles in the hip area.

Action Tips:

- Ease into a stretching routine if you're just starting out. Use legitimate guidelines for safe stretching, whether it is through a professional fitness trainer, a video of stretching exercises, or a book with clear photographs or illustrations of proper positioning

- Be sure to warm up before stretching by simply moving each joint with rotating movements to increase the synovial fluid or joint lubricant, as well as to increase the blood flow to the muscles. Keep in mind, your muscles are not always warm and supple. You might think about them as frozen chicken wings. Would you stretch the frozen wing without warming it up? If you did, chances are you would see and hear tearing of tissue. This is definitely a vision to keep in mind while stretching!

- Only hold each stretch from ten to thirty seconds. Repeat three to five times before you move on to the next stretch.

- Inhale deeply before stretching a muscle group. Gently exhale as if you were softly blowing out a candle while you move into the stretch.

- If you feel any pain during a stretch, stop! You should expect to feel a bit of discomfort as your muscles and joints begin to loosen up. Stop if you feel dizzy at any time. Sometimes dizziness occurs if you have failed to breathe throughout your stretching. Many of us have a natural tendency to tense up and stop breathing while holding each position. Relax the muscles as you stretch and be aware of your breathing.

- Avoid bouncing as this is not good for your muscle fibers. Remember the chicken wing? Your muscles appreciate a gentle, holding action. The goal of the stretch is simply to elongate the muscle fibers, to counteract their natural tendency to contract to a shorter length. The shorter the length, the less mobility one will have. When you awaken, stretch before you rise out of bed.

- Devote fifteen to twenty minutes per day to stretching. If you spend quite a bit of time sitting or standing in one position, plan on several stretch breaks during the day.

- If stretching is enjoyable to you, check out a yoga program, as stretching is a major part of this ancient form of exercise.

FMI:
Stretching by Robert A. Anderson & Jean E. Anderson,
Shelter Publications, Bolinas, California, 2000

---

*Twenty-five percent of all the oxygen in your body
is constantly being used by your brain!*

Cop an Attitude

We are the heroes of our own story.
—Mary McCarthy—

Did You Know: Roughly 30 percent of people who are given a placebo, or fake pill, to help cure a negative health condition will totally recover, despite the predicted outcome of research scientists. It turns out the only determining factor that makes these people different from their nonplacebo-responding friends was their attitude, outlook on life, and determination. Time and time again doctors have seen it in those extra-special patients, who haven't given up, even with a supposed terminal illness, and they became totally well! What a great representation of the power of the mind!

A Healthy Attitude: Though the idea of improving your health by changing your attitude may sound like a fantasy, experiments have shown that a small amount of training spread over a year can be amazingly effective. Dr. Grossarth-Maticek randomly divided 1,200 people into two groups, both of whom had scored poorly on a life outlook survey. There were two equal-sized groups of 600. The first group of 600 people were given a self-help brochure and six, one-hour training sessions spread over a one-year period. The other 600 were given no training or placebo training. When the health status of the two groups was checked thirteen years later, 409 of the people in the first group were still alive versus only ninety-seven of the equal-sized control group! If you think it's too late for you to change, think again: the average age of the people in the experiment was fifty-eight!

A Little More Evidence, Please! In the *Journal of Psychology and Aging*, a team from North Carolina State University asked 153 people of different ages to carry out memory tests after being exposed to positive and negative words to describe stereotypes about aging. Negative words included: confused, cranky, feeble, and senile, while positive words included: accomplished, active, dignified, and distinguished. Memory performance in the older adults was lower when they were primed with negative stereotypes. In contrast, there was much less difference in performance between young and older adults primed with positive stereotypes.

Attitude Items:

* A gardener was diagnosed with a terminal illness but was too busy making the world beautiful to die. He lived on!

* A woman who loses her husband to death gives up as well and dies within a few months of his departing.

* A man's favorite dog is put to sleep. The man gives up his will to live and dies shortly thereafter.

* As people get over the age of fifty, if they have a bad attitude, their health is generally worse than their more positive friends. Their memories also seem to go faster.

Attitude Maintenance: Be aware of the power of your mind. You truly are in control of your health, well-being, and life! Keep a positive attitude and surround yourself with others who have the same mindset. Those complainers want to drag everyone down with them. Be also keenly aware of your thoughts and "self-talk." Quit telling yourself "I'm bad." Start saying to yourself "I'm good." "I feel great!" "I deserve a wonderful life!" "I am grateful for all the good I have in my world!" Believe it. Feel it. Your life is a gift. Make each moment of every day count and focus upon creating joyous, happy memories.

Action Tips:

- Be an objective observer on your life. Keep track of how often you speak negatively to yourself.

- Are the people around you positive people? They should be.

- Try to dwell upon the end result of difficult tasks or situations at hand, and focus on the positive. Think about creating a great day. When you wake up in the morning, before rising, close your eyes and imagine your day as being happy and productive. Imagine people smiling at you when you smile. Connect with how you feel when you are happy. Lock in that feeling. Be grateful for the good things in your life, no matter how small. You'll become a magnet for joy.

- Read any book by Bernie S. Siegel, MD.

FMI:
101 Exercises for the Soul: A Divine Workout Plan for Body, Mind & Spirit
by Bernie Siegel, MD, New World Library, California, 2005

Fourteen thousand people die each year as a direct result
of pesticide poisoning.

Have Power over Headaches

The most frustrating thing about unwelcome and chronic pain is its mandate to revise your life. Revision marks a measure of acceptance.

—Carolyn Hardesty—

Did You Know: More than forty-five million Americans are plagued with headaches, according to the National Headache Foundation! The American Headache Society reports that every ten seconds, someone in the United States goes to the emergency room with a headache or migraine. So, if you suffer from occasional to regular headaches, you're not alone. However, many of us have accepted the fact that headaches are supposed to be a normal part of our lives and they have power over our lives. When you get a headache, life is not fun. Your job productivity probably suffers and so do your relationships with family and friends. You do not have to be controlled by headache pain.

Headache History: There are twelve types of headaches that people experience. Tension, migraine, and cluster headaches are the most common. Ninety percent of all headaches are anxiety or emotionally induced, and 98 percent of all headaches are benign. Two percent of headache sufferers might have a more serious underlying reason for headache pain and should get it checked out. Headaches are most common in women twenty to thirty years of age and men aged thirty to forty. Migraines are typically hereditary. Eighty percent of the sufferers are women, and the majority of the migraines occur one week before or during menstruation. The pain is usually characterized by a throbbing pain, located on one side of the head, in the vicinity of one eye. Some find the pain somewhat tolerable, while others might be so totally incapacitated by the pain they become nauseated, dizzy, disoriented, or experience hot flashes. Migraines can last from three hours up to three days. There is typically a neurological or hormonal predisposition to migraines. Cluster headaches got their name because they usually occur in "bunches" over a period of a few days or months and often do not recur for lengthy periods of time. Nineteen out of twenty cluster headache sufferers are men, usually twenty to fifty years in age. The pain is usually located in the eye area and usually on one side of the head and will last for approximately ten to thirty minutes and will recur later. Tension headaches are the most common, usually resulting from some sort of stressor, making the body respond in a survival mode. The "Fight or Flight" response.

The Anatomy of a Headache: Our bodies are very sensitive to stress. The reason we experience stress in the first place (see "Check Your Stress") is rooted in the survival instinct. Although we are modern human beings, our bodies still respond to stress in much the same way as they would have thousands of years ago. The purpose of the Fight or Flight response was to facilitate some type of physical action in order to survive. The response includes an increase in blood pressure, increase in adrenalin output, increase in platelet production (in order to prepare for any wounds that might be inflicted), vasoconstriction (constriction of blood vessels), and an increase in blood sugar. Talk about pent-up energy! If we can't release the energy, we experience a kind of "power surge," and we blow a fuse. Headaches are kind of like blowing a fuse. They are usually caused by an initial constriction of the blood vessels in the head, and because the brain says, "Hey, we need more oxygen up here!" there is a sudden opening of the vessels causing severe pressure—hence the headache.

A Stage Production: Headaches develop in four stages. Stage one is when positive thoughts and emotions might stop the headache in its tracks. Drugs are usually useless in stage one. However, visualizing a balloon deflating in your head and biofeedback are typically quite effective. Stage two is when the constriction of the blood vessels of the head occurs. This is also where headaches take different paths. Tension headaches go for the "band around the head" effect. In migraines, you might experience seeing stars or have other visual problems. This is called an "aura," which approximately 50 percent of migraine sufferers experience. Some feel this happens because of oxygen deprivation. In cluster headaches, no changes are evident in to the sufferer in stage two. Stage three is when the blood vessels open wide or dilate in order to provide the brain with what it desires. Unfortunately, it's overload time and severe pressure is the result. Stage four is when pain makes its debut! However, in observations of athletes injured during a game and soldiers wounded in battle, it was observed that if there are other feelings involved such as enthusiasm of winning a game or relief at leaving battle, the pain was lessened. At this stage the amount of pain you experience depends upon where your mind is!

Doctor, Doctor: You should visit your physician if you experience chronic debilitating pain; headache pain after a blow to the head; a sudden onset of severe, sharp pains in the head area; or any headache that is unusual and prevents you from performing your day-to-day tasks.

Pain Begone! There are some wonderful, new pharmaceutical drugs that work well to relieve pain. Another method to alleviate pain is to apply ice packs around the base of your neck. If cold doesn't work, try heat, especially moist heat. A hot bath might do the trick. Massage your neck muscles. Exercise. Stand and swing your arms side to side for a count of one hundred. This is a Chinese form of movement that forces the blood vessels in your hands and feet to dilate, forcing blood away from your head. Biofeedback, in which you are hooked up to a machine that monitors your skin temperature or muscle tension, might work. In one example of biofeedback you work with a computer screen that shows you a graphic. You need to reduce the graphic in size by decreasing your muscle tension. The reduction in size is your feedback, resulting in a greater awareness of your own sense of control over tension and ability to decrease the severity of headaches with "physical focus."

Feverfew herb has gotten some attention in the *British Journal of Medicine* as a possible migraine preventative. Two 50 milligram capsules were administered daily over a period of two and a half years. Thirty percent of migraine sufferers reported no more headaches, 70 percent reported fewer headaches than before, and 40 percent experienced better sleep and less muscle discomfort.

Pure oxygen inhaled by cluster headache sufferers during the onset of this type of headache seemed to arrest it immediately.

Action Tips:

- Think positively. Positive thoughts are a wonderful headache preventative. When you experience and dwell upon negative thoughts and emotions, your hypothalamus and pituitary glands think you are under stress and kick in the "fight or flight response."

- Identify your headache triggers. Common triggers are negative thoughts and emotions; high protein diets; too many processed foods containing artificial colorings, flavorings, sugar, preservatives, fat, etc.; foods that are marinated or fermented; lack of exercise; food sensitivities; environmental pollutants such as cigarette smoke, cleaning chemicals and carbon monoxide; weekend caffeine withdrawal; too much caffeine; low blood sugar; high altitudes; poor posture; premenstrual hormonal shifts; cold foods; birth control pills; flashing bright lights or too much sunlight; loud noises; and certain medications such as nitroglycerine, which causes blood vessels to dilate.

- Twenty-five to 35 percent of migraine sufferers will respond to dietary modification.

- Don't feel powerless over your headaches. Remember, knowledge is power.

FMI:
National Headache Foundation
820 N. Orleans, Suite 217
Chicago, Illinois 60610. Phone: 1-888-NHF-5552
Web: www.headaches.org

American Headache Society
19 Mantua Road
Mount Royal,
New Jersey 08061. Phone: 856-423-0043
Web: www.americanheadachesociety.org

Honey is the only food that doesn't spoil.

Get a Handle on Those "Sat-Fats"

One should eat to live, not live to eat.
—Moliere—

Did You Know: Dropping the amount of saturated fats and trans-fats you eat every day is not only a means to prevent cardiovascular disease, heart attacks, strokes, and high cholesterol, but also lessens the likelihood you'll die from cancer. Many experts believe that we need to drop our total daily consumption of fats, especially saturated fats, to less than 10 percent of our total calories! The National Cancer Institute, the National Academy of Sciences, the American Cancer Society, and the Surgeon General have all recommended we consume fats in moderation, choosing "good fats" over "bad" in order to reduce the incidence of cancer and heart disease.

Fat Facts: Most foods contain several different kinds of fat—including unsaturated, trans-fats, and saturated—and some types are better for your health than others are. It's not necessary that you completely eliminate all fats from your meals. Rather, choose the best types of fat and enjoy them in moderation.

There Are Three Major Fat Types
Unsaturated fats (Including Monounsaturated and Polyunsaturated fats): Found in plant foods and fish they may be good for heart health. The best of the unsaturated fats are found in olive oil, peanut oil, canola oil, albacore tuna, and salmon.

Trans-fats: These fats are found in margarine, especially the sticks. Trans-fats are also found in certain foods that you buy at the store or in a restaurant, such as snack foods, baked goods, and fried foods. When you see "hydrogenated" or "partially hydrogenated" oils on an ingredient list, the food contains trans-fats. Like saturated fats, eating too much can raise cholesterol and increase the risk of heart disease.

Saturated Fats: Along with trans-fats, "sat-fats" are directly responsible for the high incidence of obesity, cancer, and heart disease in this country. "Sat-fats" are stable substances and are solid at room temperature. Lard and pure butter are examples of saturated fats. You'll also find them in abundance in beef, chicken, pork, and whole milk products such as cheese, yogurt, sour cream, etc. Egg yolks contain five grams of fat per yolk, which multiplied times nine calories per gram, weighs in at forty-five calories of fat. Since the yolk probably contains 60 calories, it totals out to be approximately 80 percent fat! High levels of saturated fats in a diet are responsible for a phenomenon called "Blood Sludging." When these fats are consumed, the cells have a tendency to "clump" together, slowing the flow of oxygen-rich blood to your tissues. Do you feel energized or sleepy after a high fat meal? Point made! They also raise the level of "bad" cholesterol, hence raising your overall cholesterol count. "Sat-fats" have more impact upon your cholesterol than even high cholesterol foods.

The Scoop on Fat: Fat is a powerhouse of energy, weighing in at a hefty 9 calories per gram as compared to 4 calories per gram for both carbohydrates and protein. It doesn't take an incredible amount of energy for your body to assimilate and store away those fat calories. Carbohydrates, on the other hand, are either burned for fuel immediately or are stored away in the form of glycogen in your muscles and liver in order to be available to be used for energy later on. Protein-calories take quite a bit of energy to convert to amino acids, which are then sent to build muscle tissue, specific protein based cells, etc. Fats, especially saturated fats, contribute to your "fat pads," increase the amount of cholesterol and triglycerides in your bloodstream, contribute to the build-up of plaque inside the blood vessel walls, and increase the risk of cancer when they are "oxidized" in your bloodstream, which turns them into carcinogenic substances.

Fat and Females; Dr. John MacDougall feels the high level of fat in the typical American diet has not only contributed to the "pear-shape" phenomenon or excessive amount of fat being deposited on the hips and thighs of American women, but also that eating high amounts of fat can create a hormonal imbalance. The bottom line? Dr. MacDougall thinks PMS and early menopause may be directly linked to the high amount of "sat-fat" foods in our diets. Saturated fats help the body create more estrogen.

Action Tips: Keep a food diary (see "Be Your Own Nutritionist"). Then calculate your average daily caloric intake. Use an ideal body weight reference of a male at 5 feet 2 inches, weighing in at 118, adding 6 pounds for every inch over five-foot-two. For an ideal body weight for women, use 5 feet at 100 pounds as a base, then add 5 pounds for every inch over 5 feet. If you are a sedentary person, multiply your ideal body weight by the number eleven. Multiply by eighteen if you're extremely active. From this number, which is an estimate of your daily calories, figure what 10 percent of that number would be. This number is the number of calories you should obtain from saturated fats. Divide by 9 calories. This result is equivalent to the number of grams you should not exceed from saturated fats! How much total fat, including polyunsaturated and saturated fats, do you need? Figure 10 percent, 15 percent, and 20 percent of your calories as a baseline for your TOTAL fat calories. Choose a specific level in which you feel comfortable. The number of daily fat grams should fall into the realm of 20 to 40 grams per day for women, and 30 to 50 grams for men.

Stick to the "Fat Gram" program, and you'll not only change your affinity for fats, you'll improve your chances for living a healthy and long life.

A person who smokes one pack of cigarettes per day will inhale approximately one-half cup of tar annually.

Move It

We are not permitted to choose the frame of our destiny.
But what we put into it is ours.

—Dag Hammarskjöld—

Did You Know: Healthy human beings were designed to move. We can crawl, walk, run, jump, skip, hop, row a boat, throw a ball, roll down a hill, ice skate, climb a tree, make love, carry children, swim, surf—well, you get the picture! Most of us enter into this world as a bundle of energy, with even our toes moving as we meet our new environment! We are creatures, as many others on the earth, who move for a variety of reasons with the main one being survival. Thousands of years ago, if we couldn't move we couldn't hunt for food, procreate, or defend ourselves. You need to move your body not only to survive, but to thrive!

Not Gettin' Any Younger: As you get older and you limit your activity, your joints and muscles will respond accordingly and tighten up. If your movement is limited, your heart doesn't have to work as hard to pump oxygen-rich blood to your tissues. This results in a weaker heart muscle. Your lungs don't have to work as hard either because you don't need as much oxygen to "run" your machine, or body. As your lungs adapt to a lesser demand, their capacity to take in a maximal amount of air decreases! And the effects of lessened movement are upon you—you "feel" old!

Become Nostradamus: Would you like to see into your future? How about knowing how long you will live? When the highest-intensity aspect of exercise is measured, it has been proven to be a better predictor of how long someone will live than other factors—including health risk factors like high cholesterol, diabetes, smoking, high blood pressure, and even heart disease. Researchers from Stanford University, Veterans Affairs Palo Alto Health Care System, tested more than 6,200 men and concluded that their chances of staying alive increased by 12 percent with each increase of a single metabolic equivalent or MET. MET is used to estimate the amount of oxygen used by the body during physical activity.

The harder your body works during the activity, the higher the MET. Simply, this study shows that traditional strategies of increasing longevity does little when compared to the strategy of using exercise to improve health and fitness.

Reverse the Process! Making a concerted effort to stay active, as each year passes will make you a happier and healthier person. According to recent research, people who take a daily stroll will outlive their inactive friends. Better yet, those who engage in aerobic activities that involve getting the heart rate up to a "target level" for a period of twenty to sixty minutes three to five times per week will make their heart, lungs, muscles, and bones strong and youthful. If you exercise aerobically, which includes activities such as walking, running, stair stepping, rowing, cycling, and swimming—just to name a few. You can actually increase your good cholesterol levels, or high-density lipoproteins (HDLs). HDLs help sweep the artery-clogging bad cholesterol, or low-density lipoproteins (LDLs), out of your body! Also, the term "aerobic" literally means "with oxygen," and it is the optimal state at which your body burns fat for fuel. Resistance training, on the other hand, doesn't use as much fat for energy. Resistance does, however, increase the amount of muscle in your body, which in turn increases your body's overall ability to move fat in the long run!

A Healthy Combination: If you incorporate a good stretching program, some resistance training, as well as moderate aerobic activity in your weekly regime, you very well might discover the fountain of youth . . . and energy! In addition, if you eat optimally, with the right combination of healthful foods, you'll experience a wide variety of benefits. These include increased efficiency of your heart, improved circulation, increased blood volume, increased lung capacity, increased ability to burn fat calories, and overall increased metabolic rate. In addition, you'll have lower blood pressure, lower cholesterol, less stress, a stronger immune system, and a lesser likelihood of developing heart disease or cancer. Your sex drive will improve, you'll be less depressed, and you'll have higher self-esteem. Your blood sugar will stabilize, lessening symptoms of diabetes or hypoglycemia. You'll build and maintain your bone mass, and you'll improve your range of motion in your joints!

More Is Not Necessarily Better: To maintain health, according to the American College of Sports Medicine, working out aerobically three times per week for twenty to sixty minutes is adequate. To improve health, a regime that includes aerobic, resistance, and flexibility exercises should be performed four to five times per week. Over training will result in excess fatigue, muscle tissue breakdown, a weakened immune system, and frazzled nerves!

Action Tips:

- If you're just starting out on a "Move It" program, be sure to choose an activity you like, and take it easy.

- Stop if you feel dizzy or uncomfortable at any time.

- Begin with small increments, such as walking for ten minutes, to slowly build up your stamina. Increase the length of time each week by five or ten minutes. Stabilize your aerobic routine at between twenty and sixty minutes, three to five times per week.

- Be sure to maintain your target heart rate. But if you have trouble finding your pulse, simply monitor yourself with a "talk test." That is, during your peak aerobic activity, you should still be able to carry on a conversation without sounding completely out of breath. To find your target heart rate, use the following equation:

  (220 – your age = maximum heart rate x .6 = your minimum target range. Multiply your maximum heart rate x .8 to find your maximum target range.)

  Work within this range for an effective aerobic workout. (If you take heart or blood pressure medication, your range might be much lower than your normal target. See your physician for advice.)

- Be sure to drink one cup of pure, room-temperature water fifteen to thirty minutes before exercise. If you get hot during your aerobic workout, drink cool water every fifteen to twenty minutes while exercising. Be sure to drink plenty of water throughout the day.

- If you want to engage in group exercise classes, be sure the instructors are qualified and are certified by one of the following: American College of Sports Medicine (ACSM), ACE, or the Cooper Clinic of Dallas.

·

FMI:
American Heart Association's online fitness resource site
www.justmove.org. Includes exercise diary and other fitness resources.

*The faster the background music, the more you'll eat during
a meal; the slower it is, the less you'll eat.*

Go for the Garlic

Perseverance is not a long race; it is many short races one after another.

—Walter Elliot—

Did You Know: Garlic is one of the most powerful natural healing foods on the planet. In the ancient Egyptian papyruses, a medical journal four-thousand-years-old mentions garlic twenty-two times as a medicinal herbal remedy for a plethora of illnesses. In the ancient times, garlic was used as a remedy for intestinal disorders, flatulence, worms, respiratory infections, skin diseases, wounds, symptoms of aging, and many other ailments. Through the Middle Ages into World War II, the use of garlic to treat wounds surfaced repeatedly. It was ground up or sliced and was applied directly to wounds to inhibit the spread of infections. To date, there are more than three thousand publications from all over the world that have confirmed the recognized health benefits of garlic.

Irresistible to researchers, due to the fact that it's been around for in excess of four millennia, they couldn't help but take a closer look at what exactly makes garlic so healthful.

I've Got a Crush! Crushing garlic creates a mini chemical reaction. There are two main components found separately in the cloves. When crushed, the two components, allin and allinase, form allicin. Allicin is what you smell. It is sulfur-based, hence the scent strong enough to ward off vampires if hung around your neck. Better yet, essence of crushed garlic behind your ears might prove to be even more effective. Allicin is the primary component responsible for garlic's healing properties.

Allicin Wonderland: Ah, the wonders of garlic! Here are just a few of the benefits:

- Opens or dilates blood vessels

- Decreases cholesterol, triglycerides, and blood pressure

- Decreases rate of colon, rectal, and breast cancer

- Prevents free radical damage from radiation, chemical exposure, and food additives

- Lowers LDLs, or the "bad" cholesterol

- Prevents formation of clots by "thinning" blood, thereby preventing strokes

- Protects against liver damage, especially during chemotherapy

- Fights yeast or Candida, as well as the need for prescription drugs

- Inhibits lipoxygenase, a major promoter of tumor growth

- Prevents nitrates from converting into nitrosamines, which directly lead to cancer

Back Up Please? Garlic is acknowledged as a medicine in the United Kingdom. People who live in regions of Italy, Greece, India, and China consume large amounts of garlic and have much lower rates of stomach cancer and lower cholesterol and triglycerides.

Action Tips:

- For health enhancement, eat the equivalent of one to two cloves of garlic per day. For more impact, eat the equivalent of two to three. To have significant impact, seven to ten.

- Some people experience gas, upset stomach, etc. from too much garlic. Adjust the amount you eat to suit your system. The boost to your health from the right amount for you is based on thousands of years of clear evidence.

- Take a garlic supplement, especially if you aren't that crazy about eating the potent, healing bulb!

Hair grows at a rate of 0.00000001 mile per hour.

Tap into Clean Water

Dying is no accomplishment; we all do that.
Living is the thing.
—Red Smith—

Did You Know: Your body is made up of about 70 percent water! Water plays an integral part in almost every bodily process. It is needed for the following functions:

- Transportation of nutrients

- Assisting cell growth

- Maintaining normal body temperature

- Carrying waste products out of your body

We are constantly losing moisture through perspiration and elimination of waste. If we don't replenish our body's water supply, proper functioning is affected. Water balance is essential to optimal health. Drinking pure, clean water on a daily basis is an absolute must. You should make a conscious effort to drink eight glasses of plain water daily. Your body likes water at room temperature unless your temperature is elevated after a good workout. If you have a healthy high temperature, cool water is desirable to provide quick cooling.

Water Anyone? Not getting enough water can lead to many diseases, according to Dr. F. Batmanghelidj's book, *Your Body's Many Cries for Water*. Dr. "B" argues that "water activates your body's systems," and the lack of it causes a variety of "thirst" responses we call "disease." As a result of extensive research into the role of water in the body, the author, a medical doctor, believes he has found chronic dehydration to be the cause of many conditions including asthma, allergies, arthritis, angina, migraine headaches, hypertension, raised cholesterol, chronic fatigue syndrome, multiple sclerosis, depression, and diabetes in the elderly. Additionally, most of us are chronically dehydrated, and we have to discipline ourselves to drink water to avoid this. If you drink only when you are thirsty, it's too late—you are already dehydrated. Last, as you get older, your sense of thirst doesn't work properly.

Seek out the Clean H_2O! Finding clean water is another matter! Since the onset of chlorination of our nation's water supply in 1908, contracting bacterial and viral diseases have practically been eliminated from our water supply. The only problem is increased contamination of our great water reserves by pollutants! Industrial wastes, pesticides, fertilizers, sewage, and toxic materials in dumps have all threatened our supplies. Water can also be contaminated by lead from old lead pipes found in older neighborhoods and lead solder of copper pipes (eliminated in 1978). Natural radon might also contaminate your water, which isn't a problem in drinking, but when you turn the faucet or shower on the gas can be released into your home environment. In addition, the chemicals used to purify your tap water might be culprits in causing health problems such as high cholesterol, mottling of teeth, and cancer!

What to Do: Because there are varying levels of purity among the fifty thousand water-processing systems in this country, some water might be better quality than others. Impure water doesn't necessarily look or smell bad. It is estimated that 25 percent of gastrointestinal illnesses of tap water drinkers were caused by bacteria from the tap water, bacteria that slipped by the purification process. There has also been a variety of instances where unknowing parents were mixing infants' formula with lead-contaminated water, causing permanent damage to their children's brain functions. High nitrates in water from fertilizers are not only known to be precursors to cancer, but also might cause a rate form of anemia in infants called "blue baby syndrome."

Action Tips:

- Let your water run a few minutes before using it, especially if you haven't used it for a while.

- Test your water. Call the EPA safe drinking water hotline (800-426-4791) for labs in your area.

- Look at alternatives. Use bottled water or get more information on water treatment kits you can purchase. Also look at carbon filters, reserve osmosis filters, and other home treatment methods. In other words, think before you drink!

You are five times more likely to die from heart disease than you are from getting into an accident.

Get Juiced!

Let your food be your medicine and let your medicine be your food.
—Hippocrates—

Did You Know: One of the best ways to fight disease and enhance your health and longevity is to include plenty of nutrient-rich fresh vegetables and fruits. Many of us in this fast-paced, convenience-oriented world find our diets devoid of these healthy foods. Juicing is the extraction of juice from raw fruits and vegetables. The juices are full of disease-fighting antioxidants that are known to clean out any "free radicals" in your body. If left unchecked, these free radicals could cause the growth of cancer.

What's in a Juice? Fresh juice, made from raw vegetables and/or fruits is basically water loaded with what researchers have dubbed as "anutrients," also known as pigments, flavors, and enzymes. These "anutrients" include carotenoids, allyl sulfides, tannins, indoles, and plant steroids to name a few. In addition, there are plenty of vitamins and minerals that your body needs in order to maintain optimal health.

Who Needs It? Almost everyone could benefit from two to four ounces of fresh carrot juice per day, unless you have a specific sensitivity or allergy to carrots. The juice is loaded with beta-carotene, an antioxidant, which helps fight disease, boosts your immune system and improves your night and color vision! (See "You're Betta Off with Beta-Carotene") If you want to improve your energy, maybe a fresh vegetable "cocktail" would do just the trick because of the high concentration of the "energy nutrients" such as B vitamins and minerals. If you have a difficult time digesting high fiber fruits and veggies, try drinking the juice!

Fresh Versus Processed: What's the difference? Juices packaged in bottles or cans or stored in your freezer have typically been heated in order to prevent bacterial growth. In addition, many have on their listing of ingredients artificial additives that may be harmful to your health. And do you know how long the processed juice has been "residing" in its container?

Use "Clean" Fruits and Veggies: If you don't use organic produce that has not been sprayed with chemicals during the growing process or afterwards, you should give your "raw" buddies a bath! Use a vegetable brush and a biodegradable soap. This should remove most of the toxic residues that you don't need for optimal health!

Action Tips:

- Buy an automatic juice extractor. Check out the Juiceman II or the Phoenix AEG.

- Don't juice peels of citrus fruits, apple seeds, or pits. These contain natural toxins that are not good for you.

- In the beginning, go easy on the juice! One to two ounces is enough, and then work up to four to six ounces, one to two times per day.

- Drink more vegetable juices than fruit. Too much fruit juice can throw your blood sugar off balance!

The average height and weight of the average American woman: Almost 5′4″ and 152 pounds. Average American man: 5′9″ and 180 pounds.

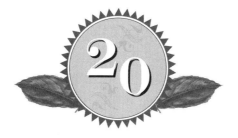

Check Your Stress

Nothing can bring you peace but yourself.
—Emerson—

Did You Know: The more people are stressed out, the less likely they are to be aware of the amount of stress they are under. The human being responds to stress, as he or she would have thousands of years ago. When survival was the name of the game, he or she either fought with or ran away from the cause of danger. For example, if you were faced with an angry, hungry saber-toothed tiger that happened to be looking at you as if you were the main course, your stress response would naturally go full throttle!

Why Don't Zebras Get Ulcers?—Or heart disease, diabetes, and other chronic diseases—when people do? According to biologist Robert Sapolsky in his book, *Why Zebras Don't Get Ulcers: An Updated Guide to Stress, Stress Related Diseases, and Coping,* people develop such diseases partly because our bodies aren't designed for the constant stresses of a modern-day life—like sitting in daily traffic jams or growing up in poverty. Rather, they seem more built for the kind of short-term stress faced by a zebra—like outrunning a lion. For example, when a lion attacks a zebra, the zebra cortisol or stress level shoots through the roof, but thereafter it returns to normal once the threat is gone. Our bodies act like we are being attacked.

Physically Speaking: Your hypothalamus, which is located at the base of your brain, is also known as the "master controller" of stress. It notifies the rest of your body to go on "full alert." In other words, get ready to fight or run! This is scientifically referred to as the "fight or flight" response. Your adrenaline output increases, which gives you abundant energy to deal with the "stressor" or immediate cause of stress!

Your heart rate increases, your breathing becomes shallow, and your blood pressure rises. Any available sugar or glucose, also known as glycogen, is released from your liver into your bloodstream to serve a source of extra energy. And to make matters a little more demanding, all of your muscles get tense, except for the muscles in your bladder and rectum . . . they relax! What would be the outcome of the hungry tiger encounter? You would probably find yourself at the top of the tallest tree around, heart racing, body on full alert, and in dire need of a restroom!

Meanwhile, in Present Time: So what happens today with this inborn mechanism to deal with stress? Your body reacts to modern-day stress the very same way it did thousands of years ago. What is different is the outcome of a stressful event. You ran from the tiger, expending a great deal of energy, using the extra adrenaline and blood sugar floating around in your system. Today, when you are stressed, you normally don't respond by getting involved in a fist fight with your boss or jogging five miles thirty minutes before you're about to get married. Remember, your reaction to stress also increases your blood pressure, heart rate, and respiration. With the number of stressors you encounter in our stress-filled society, as compared to less complicated days gone by, it is no wonder the rates of physical and emotional illness have escalated. The link between optimal health and your ability to deal with stress go hand in hand.

Stress Spells Trouble: Some people thrive on stress. Their ability to cope with a stressful event or situation might be much better than another more sensitive individual. If you are not able to nip the stress in the bud with some form of stress reduction technique, whether it is learned or innate, your immune system will suffer. Your hypothalamus, or the master controller, will continue to dictate to the rest of the body, including the adrenal glands that it is still on "alert." Your adrenal glands not only produce adrenaline, but also send out chemicals designed to repair tissues that might have been damaged in your encounter with the tiger! However, the proper functioning of your immune system is suppressed due to this "redirection" of energy. So, when you're stressed, your body's infection-fighting capabilities are lowered. Fortunately, many physicians and health professionals are beginning to acknowledge the stress and illness connection.

A Stressed Out Body: Higher and more prolonged levels of cortisol in the bloodstream (like those associated with chronic stress) have been shown to have negative physical effects too! Your body has been impacted by stress when:

- You have impaired cognitive performance or just plain "thinking." Your memory and mental clarity are affected, too.

- You show symptoms of a sluggish thyroid, cold feet, impaired thinking, weight gain, decreased libido, low energy, etc.

- Your blood sugar becomes imbalanced, with either hypo-glycemia or hyperglycemia.

- Your bone density is decreased, making your bones more susceptible to fracture.

- You have a decrease in muscle tissue or lean body mass. When you lose muscle, your metabolic rate slows down.

- You experience higher blood pressure than normal.

- You become ill more often. Stress lowers immunity and inflammatory responses in the body

- Your belly fat increases. Some of the health problems associated with increased stomach fat are heart attacks, strokes, the development of higher levels of "bad" cholesterol (LDL) and lower levels of "good" cholesterol (HDL), which can lead to other health problems.

What Do You Do? Find out how stressed out you really are. Remember, many of us are unaware of the amount of stress we are under. To be overly stressed in our society is considered normal! Rate yourself on the Holmes-Rahe Scale. According to the physicians who developed the scale, the higher your points associated with each stressful life event, the more prone you are to having your health compromised. Your health outcome, however, is also dependent upon your "coping style" and personality.

The Holmes-Rahe Scale

Scoring over three hundred points in one year greatly increases the risk of illness. A score of 150–299 reduces the risk by 30 percent, while a score of less than 150 involves a slight chance of illness. But illness is not an inevitable result of change. Your personality and your ability to cope largely determine how well you react.

Life Event	Lifechange units
Death of spouse	100
Divorce	73
Marital separation	65

Action Tips:

- Take the Holmes-Rahe Test.

- Exercise daily. People who exercise moderately are more physically able to deal with stress than those who don't work out.

- Check out relaxation techniques such as meditation, yoga, and biofeedback, and incorporate them into your daily life.

- Get an aromatherapy massage.

- Take five-minute "breathing" breaks and "laugh it off."

- Try to relax!

- See "Be Scentsible" and "Laugh It Off."

- Buy a fish bowl or tank. Sit and watch your fish and do nothing else for ten minutes. If you're a fish novice, start with freshwater fish. Your saltwater buddies dying might increase your stress level!

- Listen to a recording of the ocean. Close your eyes, trying to visualize your ideal beach (and your ideal companion). Feel the warmth of the sun on your skin, the breeze, and salty air; hear the seagulls; take yourself there.

- Drink chamomile tea. Do nothing else, except breathe. (You can drink the tea while watching your new fish.)

- Listen to soothing music—and don't try to somehow rationalize that Metallica calms you down! You know what I mean when I say soothing music—something that would make a baby sleep more restfully, not wake her up and into some sort of auditory hell on earth!

- Do simple muscle relaxation by clenching your muscles as hard as you can in each part of your body. Start with your feet, legs, buttocks, arms, shoulders, and face. Be sure your door is closed when you "clench"; then release it all.

- Take a break! Jump for five minutes on a mini-trampoline as an energizer, destressor, and lymphatic system stimulant. (Don't drink your chamomile tea while on the mini-tramp; the balancing act might stress you out!)

- Drink a cool beverage through a straw. Don't ask questions, just do it! You'll feel the benefits.

- Close your eyes and think of a number. Repeat it over and over again until your mind is blank except for the repetition of the sound of the word. Your troubles will drift away for a while.

- Imagine the air you're breathing to be blue/green. Visualize the soothing blue/green color slipping in and out of your respiratory system.

- Slice an apple in sections. Eat each section slowly, concentrating on each bite. Remember, stress relief is illness prevention. Don't think of it as just involving quality of life—it affects life itself!

Fresh fruits and vegetables lose a full 2 percent of their vitamin C content daily.

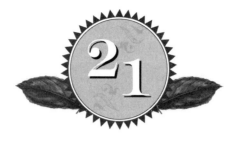

Be Balanced

If you obey all the rules you miss all the fun.
—Katharine Hepburn—

Did You Know: It really is okay to break the rules every now and then. As a matter of fact, if you take all the pleasure out of your life, what is there to enjoy? Therefore, the solution is to become a moderate extremist!

A Moderate Extremist? That's an individual who steps outside the normal realm of average effort and takes it to the fringe of the "extreme" . . . without going overboard! If you desire to have optimal health and longevity, it's best to take things gradually, perhaps making one change as each week comes along. During the first phase of your journey toward optimal health, you might want to work on dropping your fat intake. The next week, focus upon substituting "good" fats for "bad" fats in your diet. Relaxation and stretching might be your next step, and so on. However, how doesn't one fit having fun into this newly-acquired optimal health lifestyle?

The Balancing Act: It's been proven that you can actually improve your health by eating a low-fat diet, rich in whole grains, fruits, and vegetables, and moderate in protein. You can also exercise regularly, practice stress reduction techniques, and have a positive attitude to have even more of an optimal impact physically, emotionally, and mentally! But where do the hot dogs at the baseball game fit? Or the hot fudge sundaes on a summer evening? And roast beef and mashed potatoes at your mom's house?

The "Treat" Plan: Many people are eating way too many "feel good" foods and acting as if they're training for the "couch potato" Olympics! To make a significant impact on your life, you have to make up your mind that you're going to maintain a healthier lifestyle. Along with this lifestyle, you might also include "treat days" and "sloth" days, even if your doctor has told you to get your cholesterol and blood pressure down, or else! There is something to be said for enjoying life's little pleasures. Just don't enjoy them every day, every hour, or every other hour, for that manner! Giving up your cream-filled doughnut or plain bagel laden with real cream cheese that you have every morning might be a tough task. But what about just having it on Sunday morning? If you're an ice cream sundae lover, how about on Saturday afternoons?

You just have to be sure you can handle these "treats" in such a way that they don't make you fall back into your old ways! Your body will reward you with improved health and increased energy!

Watch Out for Triggers: Some people literally cannot have a high-sugar snack on occasion in the beginning stages of a new program. The sugar might trigger them to go on an eating rampage, which would not exactly be the most optimal thing that could happen. There is a biochemical connection to cravings that affect some more than others. Genetic predisposition, lack of exercise, depression, or poor nutritional status might also increase cravings. You'll find as you get your health moving in an optimal direction that your appetite will become more "normal." If you are a binge eater, you should make contact with a health professional that specializes in compulsive eating.

The Bottom Line: Make your best effort. Focus upon how great you'll look and feel, not only a few weeks from now but also ten years into the future! Being a "moderate extremist," along with eating well, staying active, and maintaining a positive attitude, might put the fountain of youth within your grasp!

Action Tips:

- Remember to be a "moderate extremist." Still experience the "fun" in life without going overboard into the "feel good" realm . . . of eating that is! You can be happy without immersing yourself in ice cream every day!

- Say to yourself, "I am a healthy eater! Being fit and healthy comes easily to me." Write it down. Place it on your refrigerator.

- "If at first you don't succeed, try, try again!"

- Know that you can do this and feel it in your heart. You deserve the best, to feel the best, to look the best, and to be happy!

In one study, women over sixty, who drank one cup of coffee per day, were more sexually active than those who didn't drink coffee. Coffee-drinking men were also more "active" and had fewer problems with intimacy!

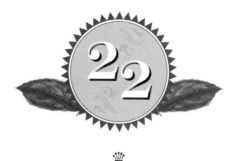

Be a Restaurant Survivor

Groan and forget it!

—Jessamyn West—

Did You Know: Too many Americans have chosen unhealthy lifestyle habits, such as not exercising, drinking too much alcohol, smoking cigarettes, and eating way too many high-fat foods. Food in restaurants is predominately geared toward the typical American's palate. And many of us fall victim to the scenario of becoming a mindless diner! If your desire is to get healthy and look and feel better, then, by using a few tricks, it'll be a piece of cake to take control of your eating in the "restaurant zone."

Tips for "Mindful" Dining: These tips are assuming you are not in the "moderate extremist" mode, desiring a weekly "treat" experience!

- Choose your restaurant carefully! Be realistic! "Granny's Fried Chicken House" usually cannot fulfill healthy diner's needs. Don't make yourself out to be a victim of circumstances.

- Have a positive attitude when dealing with your waiter or waitress. Explain what you would desire in a concise and friendly manner.

- Look for the key words, such as baked, poached, grilled, or broiled. Ask that no extra added fat be used in cooking.

- Have the skin removed from your chicken, Cornish hen, or turkey before it's cooked.

- Request all extra fat such as butter, margarine, oil, cream, sauces, mayonnaise, egg yolks, and cheese not be included in your entrée. Of course, if you order Lobster Thermador, which is floating in cream sauce, this might be an unrealistic request.

- Put on your "healthy blinders" and only focus upon the basics. Order baked salmon (hold the cream sauce and butter). Or try a baked, skinless chicken breast seasoned with herbs, such as rosemary.

- Avoid all fried foods, anything with cream sauce, and red meat.

- Call ahead to make a special request. Most chefs are accommodating and will grant your "healthy wishes."

- Double up on your carbohydrates. Keep your protein intake down to a reasonable level, depending upon how much you've eaten up to that point during the day. If it's a lunch meal, and you have animal protein, remember to keep the portion small if you're going to have some at dinner as well. Or make your evening meal vegetarian.

- In Italian restaurants, stick with ordering red sauce or plain marinara on your pasta. Pasta primavera is an excellent pasta dish, usually in a red sauce, loaded with healthy vegetables. Order vegetarian pizza without cheese. Have fruit or Italian ice for dessert.

- Limit your alcohol intake to one to two glasses of wine, in a "treat" setting. If alcoholism runs in your family, drink carbonated water with a wedge of lime instead. Why repeat a pattern?

- Chinese: Choose items that have been steamed, boiled, or broiled. Specify no oil. Avoid fried noodles. Regular boiled noodles are fine.

- Mexican food lovers can load up on fresh vegetables dipped in salsa. Chicken fajitas, rice, and beans (not refried), steamed corn tortillas, gazpacho, and green salads can all be ordered at most any Mexican restaurant.

- For fast food "victims" . . . dry baked potatoes, chicken sandwiches without the sauce, a green salad with a squeeze of lemon, and iced tea or water instead of soft drinks or "deadly" shakes!

"High Flying": Pack your own! In this day and age of minimal food service in the air, the "safest" strategy is to simply pack your own low-fat, healthy snack or meal. Always be prepared for delays and pack extra items. Blanched almonds are an excellent protein snack, will keep your blood sugar within the normal range, and supply "good" fat and fiber. Drink plenty of water while flying!

The Dining Experience: Enjoy eating out for the social experience. Focus on the ambiance and savor your surroundings. Take the focus off of food and your stomach! Enjoy the process of slowly savoring each and every bite of food.

Action Tips:

- Become comfortable with special ordering.

- Plan ahead, keeping in mind your night out throughout the day, and balance foods accordingly. Eat less fat during the day than you usually do.

- Stay aware of your needs and desires, preventing yourself from making your restaurant visit a mindless experience!

What is the percentage of Americans who die in health care institutions? A frightening 80 percent.

Balance Your Moods
With Foods

Where there is an open mind, there will always be a frontier.
—Charles F. Kettering—

Did You Know: What you eat might affect how happy or depressed you are. How about the idea of having an impact upon your level of alertness? Dr. Eric Braverman, former Chief Clinical Researcher at the Princeton Brain Bio Center, a leading figure in the practice of brain-body health care, believes that proper brain nutrition can have an effect on the quality of our lives. The key to longevity and well-being, according to Dr. Braverman, is balancing the brain's four important neurotransmitters, which, in turn, can reverse or prevent the debilitating effects of aging, including memory loss, weight gain, sexual dysfunction, and Alzheimer's. Scientists are proving that what's in the foods you eat can effect the chemical composition of your brain. The foods you eat can affect your mood, including your level of alertness and your perception of pain. Your thinking and feeling processes are influenced by the presence or absence of certain types of chemicals that are specific to your brain and nervous system. You parents, through their combined gene "donation" have set you up to be a biochemically unique individual. You may have a brain that is highly resilient to stress. Perhaps you thrive upon a chaotic lifestyle and end up sleeping like a baby at night! Or you may be so sensitive that drinking one cup of coffee may throw you through a loop!

The Fabulous Three: There are three brain chemicals that influence your thoughts and feelings. They are dopamine, norepinephrine, and serotonin. Foods high in protein supply the brain with significant amounts of the amino acid tyrosine. When protein foods are eaten, tyrosine moves right in and converts to the chemicals known to enhance alertness, dopamine and norepinephrine. High protein foods increase the levels of all these amino acids and decrease the synthesis of serotonin in the brain. Good protein sources include meat, chicken, fish, nuts, soy products, eggs, and dairy products.

When carbohydrates are eaten alone, tryptophan is introduced to the brain and serotonin. The calming brain chemical floods the gates, resulting in a general feeling of relaxation. Serotonin is a neurotransmitter that has the effect of reducing pain, decreasing appetite, and producing a sense of calm, and in too large a quantity, inducing sleep. If by chance you eat a high protein food at the same meal as a high carbohydrate food, the protein amino acids "muscle out" the calming chemicals resulting in a stimulated state! Healthy carbohydrate foods to turn to for anti-stress includes whole grain breads and crackers, whole grain pasta, rice, cereal, and fruits.

Your Brain: Up Close and Personal!

- Proteins keep the calming chemical, serotonin, from doing its relaxing job!

- If you have trouble with drowsiness after lunch, eat a meal high in lean protein and complex carbohydrates and low in extra fat. Also, keep your portions small.

- Ever notice you crave sweets when you're depressed? Low levels of serotonin will cause intense food cravings. Your brain is trying to self-medicate and raise serotonin levels.

- The desire to take a siesta or nap in the middle of the afternoon is a direct result of your body's biorhythms. You can fight it by drinking a small amount of caffeine and snacking on a low-fat carbohydrate snack, such as air-popped popcorn!

- Eating a high carbohydrate meal will negatively affect your performance. You'll be less alert and make more mistakes, so save it for dinner if you're going to spend a nice quiet evening at home!

Action Tips:

- Keep a daily record of what you eat throughout the day and how you feel mentally, emotionally, and physically. Continue the record for a seven- to fourteen-day period until you have a general feel as to what types of meals or snacks make you feel particularly alert, and those that seemingly have a sedative effect.

- Utilize information listed above to effectively manipulate your brain chemistry! Keep in mind the manipulation of neurotransmitters or brain chemicals is independent of moods that may be altered by blood sugar highs and lows, caused by low blood sugar or diabetes-type symptoms.

FMI:

Managing Your Mind and Mood Through Food, Judith Wurtman, PhD, Harper and Row Publishers, New York, 1988

The Edge Effect: Achieve Total Health and Longevity with the Balanced Brain Advantage, Eric R. Braverman, MD

Over 60 percent of the American population has some type of problem with their vision.

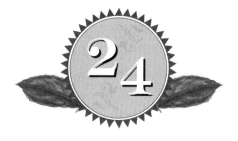

Be a "Super" Market Shopper

*Eat regularly, for an empty stomach is not
a good political advisor.*

—Unknown—

Did You Know: One of the easiest ways to get you and your family healthy is to change the way you shop at your local grocery store. As the primary shopper, whether you're single or married, you can truly make a tremendous impact upon your health if the correct focus is found in the market. Here are some basic rules to follow to get your cart lookin' healthy:

- Make a list before you go to the store. Impulse buying and lack of direction will surely set you up for some mindless purchases. Plus, you'll be more likely to stay within your budget with a list. Organize your list by sections–dairy, seafood, breads, condiments, produce, etc.

- Put those imaginary blinders on. Focus only on the items you are looking for, not on items you're not interested in! This will allow you to be "blind" to highly processed and sugar and fat-laden foods that will ultimately sabotage your health if consumed too often!

- Focus on whole grains. Avoid anything with enriched wheat flour as the primary ingredient. This is simply an impressive synonym for white, highly processed flour. You need to focus on nutritious, fiber-rich whole-grain products. Bread's first ingredient should be "100 percent whole grain or wheat." If you're looking for fat-free breads, French and Italian are nice on occasion, however, they are not as wholesome as whole-grain breads. Other whole grains include brown rice, corn tortillas (not fried), barley, legumes or beans such as lentils, split peas, black-eyed peas, pinto and black beans, tabouli, whole-wheat pasta, and whole-grain cookies.

- In the meat, poultry, and seafood section, focus mainly on low in saturated fat items such as chicken or turkey without the skin. If you desire ground poultry, have the butcher grind it for you without the skin, which they usually add for "flavor." Flank steak is a very lean cut of beef, so it requires a tenderizer before cooking. Fish containing good fats, alias omega-3s, are excellent for decreasing bad cholesterol and blood pressure. Many types of fish supply omega-3s. Salmon, tuna, halibut, and swordfish are the most optimal sources. This type of fat is essential for proper hormone production and maintaining optimum health.

- When reading labels, be sure you can pronounce most if not all of the ingredients. If the listing looks like something from your high school chemistry book, look for an alternative. With the number of deaths from cancer having risen from one in twenty, at the beginning of this century, to one in four now, it's probably a wise idea to have most of the foods you consume on a daily basis to be "clean," or without too many questionable additives. We have enough to deal with in the air we breathe!

- Go for "real" food. Low-fat and trans-fat-free items are optimal if they supply some form of good nutrition such as in a whole-grain cookie. Eating foods without fats or fat substitutes will acclimate your taste buds (it takes approximately six months to get over a love affair with fats) to a true low-fat mode. Eating foods low in fat on a daily basis will allow you to have a really great fat-filled dessert or another type of food on occasion without compromising your percentage of body fat or your long-term health!

- Make a trip to the produce section a major priority! Load up on plenty of fiber- and nutrient-rich fruits and vegetables. Focus on the more colorful fare loaded with antioxidants. Carrots, cantaloupe, and sweet potatoes are loaded with beta-carotene. Dark-green leafy vegetables such as kale, broccoli, and collard and turnip greens are high in calcium. Apples, raspberries, strawberries, and pears are excellent sources of fiber. Potatoes, oranges, lemons, and grapefruit are rich in C. Garlic and onions are the great flavor enhancers that have also been found to lower blood pressure and cholesterol as well as decrease risk of certain types of cancer!

- With the new Nutrition Labeling act now in effect, most foods will have consistent labeling information, with the added bonus of telling you what percentage of fat is in each serving, with 30 percent being the maximum acceptable guideline. Some single-ingredient raw poultry and meat products are exempt. Be sure if the label on a meat product states "97 percent fat free" to be aware they are not talking about percentage of calories. The meat product is 3 percent by weight! To calculate the true percentage of calories use the following formula: *Number of fat grams per serving x 9 calories, divided by the total number of calories per serving x 100 = percentage of calories from fat.*

  Typically, the percentage is much higher than you thought, so don't be fooled by those meats!

- Only buy oils that contain monounsaturates, with virgin olive or canola oil providing the heaviest hit of these heart-healthy fats! Saturated fats such as those found in palm kernel oil and lard raise "bad" cholesterol. Partially hydrogenated fats (read the label!) contain trans-fats, which also raise cholesterol! Best bet? Use small amounts of unsalted butter if you can't live without it! For flavor on your vegetables, try a butter spray. These are typically nonfat but still contain that buttery flavor that can enhance flavor of even the healthiest vegetables!

Almost twenty-five million Americans go under the surgeon's knife each year as a result of "unhealthy" lifestyles!

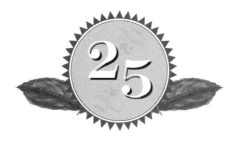

Don't Be a Smoking Gun

(Definition) "Habit, n. A shackle for the free."
—Ambrose Bierce—

Did You Know: If you smoke cigarettes, your chances of dying of a heart attack are double those of a nonsmoker. You are also two to three times more likely to have a stroke. A stroke occurs when the blood supply is partially or wholly cut off from the brain for a period of time and, nine times out of ten, is caused by clogging of the arteries in the neck. People who smoke have a higher tendency to develop these types of blockages than nonsmokers. Many people die from the stroke, while others survive. The survivors are usually permanently incapacitated in some way. The unfortunate side to smoking is that many find it pleasurable, psychologically and physiologically gratifying, due to nicotine's stimulatory effects. The bottom line is that it is so addictive physically and behaviorally that it is one of the most difficult habits to kick!

Smokin' Facts!

- Each cigarette steals away eight minutes of life.

- One pack of cigarettes per day equates to losing a month of life each year, and two packs per day means ten to twelve years off the life expectancy of lifetime smokers.

- Just one cigarette can increase the heart rate twenty to twenty-five beats per minute and can significantly increase blood pressure.

- Cigarettes contain approximately 4,000 known toxic poisons.

- Smoking a pack of cigarettes daily depletes 500 milligram of vitamin C, more than most people ingest in one day.

- Cigarettes increase carbon monoxide levels in the blood, which compete with oxygen so thoroughly that it takes the circulatory system six hours to return to normal after smoking one single cigarette.

- Smoking can be so immunosuppressive that it takes three months to reverse its damage to your immune system.

Smokers "Benefits": If you smoke, you aren't going to feel as great as you would feel as a nonsmoker. Your breathing will be labored and make you much more likely to develop breathing diseases such as lung cancer and emphysema! Your

HDLs, or good cholesterol, will be lower than nonsmokers. And the "benefit" for your friends and family who sit around and breathe in your secondary cigarette smoke is that their HDLs will lower, too! And if you smoke and try to exercise, you are more likely to suffer from mild to severe leg cramps. Best of all, cigarette smoking will mask angina, pain in the heart area. This is not a good thing, because angina is often an indicator of heart disease. Finally, if you're a man and your sex life is a little dull, consider the fact that the smoking habit and impotence are related. Apparently, smoking regularly might cause small blockages in the blood supply to the penis. Are you ready to go cold turkey?

Motivation to Give Up: According to the American Cancer Society, quitting cigarettes has immediate physical benefits, besides giving you a few more dollars to spend.

- Twenty minutes after your last cigarette:
  Your blood pressure and pulse rate drop
  to normal, and;
  The temperature of your hands and feet
  increases to normal.

- Within eight hours:
  The oxygen level in your bloodstream increases
  to normal, and;
  The toxic carbon monoxide drops to normal.

- Within twenty-four hours:
  Your chances of heart attack begin to decrease.

- Within forty-eight hours:
  Your senses of smell and taste are enhanced,
  Your nerve endings begin to regrow, and;
  Your chances of having a heart attack are decreased
  by 50 percent.

- Within seventy-two hours:
  You'll breathe easier because the bronchial tubes in
  your lungs relax.

- Within two weeks to three months:
  Your lung function increases by 30 percent, and;
  Blood circulation improves, and even walking
  becomes easier.

- All things considered, quitting smoking will decrease
  the risk of cancers (including lung cancer), stroke, and
  heart attack. Pregnant women who quit before or in the
  beginning of their pregnancy will be less likely to have
  low-birth-weight, high-risk babies.

True or False? Smoking low-tar and low-nicotine cigarettes
guarantees the smoker of being less likely to die of heart attacks
than those who smoke stronger brands. False! It doesn't matter what the "rating" is. Researchers have found absolutely no
difference in blood nicotine levels between strong brand and

weak brand users! You still are at the same risk of dying of a heart attack or cancer as an avid smoker of stronger brands!

The "Kickoff": It literally takes two weeks for nicotine to be completely removed from your body after smoking your last cigarette. So if you decide to taper down slowly you are still giving your body the addictive "feel good" substance, from which eventually you are going to have to withdraw. Going cold turkey works well for many people while others like to take it slowly. To taper down, under the supervision of a physician, getting your nicotine "fix" from the new nicotine gum or skin patches is much more desirable than continuing the destruction of your lungs and body from the smoke itself! Some former smokers claim using programs such as hypnosis and acupuncture assist in the withdrawal states. Exercise and a balanced diet also help the process along. If you're craving a cigarette, chew gum, take a walk, or munch on carrot or celery sticks. Once you've gotten over your chemical dependency on nicotine, all you have to do is get over your behavioral and psychological addiction to the habit. And if you are a pack-a-day smoker, you literally take seventy thousand puffs a year . . . or one million puffs over a twenty-year time period. If you are a smoker and you kick the habit, you truly will live a longer, healthier life!

The Power of Green: Japanese smoke more cigarettes than Americans do but have a lower incidence of cancer and heart disease. One of the protective factors in the Japanese diet is green tea. Researchers at the University of Arizona tested 140 smokers to see if drinking tea reduces the risks of cancer. They examined whether tea repaired damage to cells caused by smoking. In particular, they looked at the affects on a chemical called 8-OhDG, which is found in urine and is believed to cause cell damage.

For four months, volunteers drank green tea, black tea, or water. Only the subjects who drank green tea had a 25 percent reduction in 8-OhDG. However, no changes were seen in the people who drank black tea or water.

The polyphenols found in green tea appear to block the formation of certain cancers. This does not give you the "A-OK" to smoke; however if you can't kick the habit, supplementing with green tea may reduce some of the damaging effects of smoking.

FMI:

The American Cancer Society

Phone: 1-800-ACS-2345 Web: www.cancer.org

A nerve impulse travels at the speed of light.

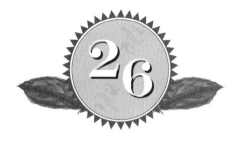

Get Energized
With Carbohydrates

*You have to learn the rules of the game.
And then you have to play better than anyone else.*

—Dianne Feinstein—

Did You Know: Carbohydrates are *the* source of quick energy in your diet! In an optimal longevity diet, your total daily calories should be divided among the three primary food sources: 10 to 15 percent protein, 30 percent fat (with 10 percent of those fat calories or less from saturated fats), and 55 to 70 percent carbohydrates. Carbs pack a mean punch when it comes to providing energy to your cells. They provide 4 calories per gram and are generally loaded with valuable vitamins, minerals, and fiber. Eating enough carbohydrates on a daily basis is essential in order to "spare" protein you've eaten so it can be used for muscle, tissue, and cellular repair and not be burned for energy. Your body will burn up valuable protein if you are not getting enough carbs. If you have low energy and have avoided carbohydrates because you thought they would make you fat, chances are you need to eat more! Eating a generous amount of complex carbohydrates will not make you fat. Eating fatty, nonnutritious foods will!

A Chain Gang: Carbohydrates are basically short and long chains of energy-containing molecules called glucose, which are actually simple sugars. The name of each type of carbohydrate depends directly upon the organization of the energy molecules. Complex carbs typically are rather long, complex chains of glucose, usually combined with some type of fiber that slows the release of glucose into your blood stream. Complex carbs are found in whole grains like whole wheat or rye, spelt, quinoa, steel-cut oats, and brown rice. They're also found in starchy vegetables such as sweet potatoes, potatoes, corn, peas, and legumes. Simple carbohydrates are usually found in refined, highly processed foods such as white flour. The valuable bran and nutrients have been removed. White or refined sugar is a straight, simple carbohydrate. When you eat simple carbs, glucose blasts into your bloodstream briskly, due to the lack of fiber. Your blood sugar will usually rise quickly. The glucose is then transported to all different parts of your body to be used as immediate energy, with some leftovers. Some are converted to glycogen—the stored carbohydrate in muscle. The rest gets converted to fluffy, greasy fat.

Don't Keep It Simple: If the majority of carbohydrates you consume come from highly processed sources such as those primarily comprised of white flour and/or white sugar, you will not be getting the vitamins, minerals, and fiber that you need to keep you healthy. The lack of fiber will predispose you to all sorts of problems (See "Fiber Your Life"), including obesity, constipation, and other digestive disorders and might also lead to many forms of cancer, such as colon and rectal cancer! Because you need certain vitamins and minerals to assimilate carbohydrates in general, and refined carbs usually provide less than optimal nutrition, you'll be drawing from your own body's stores of nutrients in order to metabolize the simple sugar. Say hello to nutrient debt!

Do Carbs Make You Fat? Some experts point out that if all carbohydrates were responsible for obesity, countries that consume the greatest amount of carbs as a percentage of calories in their diet, would suffer the most. Yet this is not the case. Residents of third world countries, who tend to consume less protein and fat in their diet, are relatively unscathed by obesity. Also, in Japan, carbohydrates compose the majority of daily caloric intake. High carb foods like grains, rice, and vegetables are daily staples of the Japanese diet, and intake of high-protein, high-fat animal products is minimal. In contrast to the "horrors" of carbohydrates as described by promoters of some almost-no-carb diets, Japan has one of the lowest rates of obesity, heart disease, cancer, and diabetes in the world. This indicates the types of carbs eaten can have dramatic effects on health.

Be a Complex Individual: Eating a diet rich in grains and starchy vegetables will provide you with an abundance of complex carbohydrates. Try to get at least six servings per day if you're a lightly active female and up to eleven servings if you're a male athlete! One serving is one-half cup cooked cereal such as steel-cut oats, one-half cup of brown rice or whole-wheat pasta (white pasta is a great source of energy filled carbs, but low in fiber), one slice of whole-grain bread, one-half cup of pinto beans, or one small potato.

A Fruity Concept: How does fruit fit into this scenario? Fruit is rich in a more simple sugar called fructose or fruit sugar. Fructose typically has a gentle impact upon blood sugar and, in the form of high fiber fruits, provides an ideal route for quick, nutritious carbohydrate calories. Two to four servings of whole fruits are recommended over and above the complex carbohydrate recommendations.

Action Tips:

- Switch to whole-grain breads, pastas, brown rice, tortillas, and pass up their refined cousins. Consume at least half of your carbohydrates from whole grain sources.

- Be sure to obtain a minimum of six servings per day to eleven maximum.

- Calculate your daily caloric intake, and figure 55 to 70 percent of those carbohydrate calories.

- Don't eat refined, sugary foods every day. Use them as treats, for special occasions, or on a weekly, designated treat day.

Women eat more under stress, whereas men eat less!

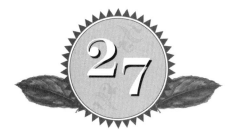

Boost Your Brain Power
with Blueberries

What a wonderful life I've had!
I only wish I'd realized it sooner!
—Colette—

Did You Know: Blueberries are special. Those delicious yet delicate berries happen to pack a huge punch with it comes to your brain. The United States Department of Agriculture (USDA) tested twenty-four varieties of fresh fruit, twenty-three fresh vegetables, sixteen herbs and spices, ten different nuts, and four dried fruits. They found blueberries scored the highest in overall total antioxidants per serving. Anthocynanins (the reason why blueberries are blue!) and their precursor, proanthocynaidins are abundant in this tiny powerhouse. These antioxidants are responsible for countering free radicals, the harmful byproducts of cellular metabolism that can contribute to cancer, heart disease, cognitive decline, and other age-related diseases.

The Brain Game: Your brain is highly metabolic, no different than other organs you have, and it suffers from free radical damage. Some scientists believe that age-related decline in mental function is due to a lifetime of free radical hits to your brain. In a *Journal of Neuroscience* study, one group of rats were fed the equivalent of one half cup of blueberries per day. In other groups, rats were given food extracts such as spinach, strawberries, and a "control" diet low in antioxidants. Once the rats reached the age equivalent of seventy to seventy-five-year-old humans, they were given various memory function tests. All of the groups outperformed the "control" diet-fed rats. Blueberry fed rats were the champions, significantly outperforming the other groups.

An Intelligent Destination: Blueberries have been shown to cross the blood brain barrier much like alcohol does. The blood brain barrier is semi-permeable and allows some materials but prevents others from crossing. What is the blood brain barrier? The blood brain barrier is semi-permeable. It allows some materials to cross, but prevents others from making the journey through to the brain. Alcohol readily crosses the blood-brain barrier, which causes rapid effects. Examining the brains of rats that had been fed blueberry extract for ten weeks, researchers were able to isolate blueberry-specific agents in the rats' cerebellum, cortex, hippocampus, and striatum—brain areas that control memory and learning processes. Blueberry phytochemicals were found to be present in the areas of the rat's brains associated with cognitive performance. This correlation between blueberries and improved memory and learning makes this sweet fruit a powerful brain booster!

Action Tips:

The key to preventing cognitive decline is to keep your brain active. The Institute for the Study of Aging and the International Longevity Center-USA recommend the following strategies to keep your mind functioning as effectively as possible as you age:

- Have at least one cup of blueberries a day.

- Stay socially active. A study published in the August 1999 issue of the *Annals of Internal Medicine* found that having no social ties was an independent risk factor for cognitive decline in older persons.

- Keep learning. Many studies on humans and animals suggest that lifelong learning is beneficial in preserving cognitive vitality in later life. One such study, published in the February 2002 issue of the *Journal of the American Medical Association,* found that frequent participation in mentally stimulating activities is associated with a reduced risk of Alzheimer's disease.

- Mental stimulation is not limited to formal education and can include everyday activities such as:

— Reading books, newspapers, or magazines

— Playing games such as:
  o   Cards
  o   Checkers
  o   Crosswords or other puzzles
  o   Going to museums

— Exercise—Studies show improved cognitive functioning in older adults who exercise. Exercise may contribute to cognitive vitality by improving mood and reducing stress and other risk factors that contribute to decline in memory and learning as you age.

Heart attacks are more likely to occur in the middle of the day rather than in the morning. Monday is by far the leading day of the week for heart attacks.

Take a Walk

The quality of a life is determined by its activities.
—Aristotle—

Did You Know: Walking is the number one exercise in the United States. If done on a regular basis, a person might actually decrease high blood pressure, lower his resting heart rate, lessen the risk of stroke or heart attack, raise HDL or good cholesterol levels, lower body fat, increase metabolism, strengthen bones and muscles, and have increased energy and stamina! Not bad for doing something we were naturally designed to do on a regular basis.

The Big Payoff: If you want to live a longer and healthier life, start now with daily walking or exercise. A study in the November 14, 2005, "Archives of Internal Medicine" showed that exercise levels are directly related to years lived without cardiovascular disease. A moderate level of physical activity, such as walking thirty minutes a day, lengthened life by 1.3 years and added 1.1 more years without cardiovascular disease, compared with those with low activity levels. Those who chose a high physical activity level gained 3.7 years of life and added 3.3 more years without cardiovascular disease. An editorial in the "Washington Post" did the math—invest thirty minutes of walking a day and you'll spend forty-nine days of the next twelve years of your life walking to gain 1.3 healthy years. That's a great payoff, considering that it is also likely the walking will help you decrease your body fat and improve your mood.

Move It! Our bodies need exercise to stay healthy. By moving around, we automatically place a "good" type of stress upon our muscles and bones, which strengthens them. However, the way you move about is also important.

- **Get in Line!** The way you hold and execute your body in space is of ultimate importance for walking. Even the most enthusiastic walker might suffer from discomfort and even injuries if proper body alignment techniques aren't used. Follow these guidelines. Begin by standing with your feet parallel and place your weight back toward your heels, placing your shoulders directly above your hips. Hold your abdominals tight, keep your head directly on top of your spine, and keep your chin level. Imagine a string pulling you up through the crown of your head in order to lengthen your spine.

- **One Step at a Time:** When you step forward, be sure to roll heel to toe, keeping your knees in line with the center of your feet. As you step, become aware of each muscle group involved. Lightly squeezing your buttock muscles as you step through can help tone and strengthen your entire hip area. Become aware of your inner thigh muscles as well. Make them work, too! Your arms should be relaxed and swing naturally as you walk. If you choose a very brisk pace, your arms should be bent, kept close to your body, and moved forward and back, not side to side.

- **How Fast?** Your pace is going to totally depend upon your present level of fitness. If the pace you choose leaves you breathless, slow down. You should be able to carry on a conversation easily. Fitness walkers usually choose a pace between fourteen and eighteen minutes per mile. A twelve- to fifteen-minute mile can give the same physical and psychological benefits as jogging. Fitness experts recommend to vary your pace and intensity for maximal cardiovascular benefits. The good old "walk, jog, walk" technique does have its advantages! If you're just a stroller, you'll still increase your life expectancy over and above your inactive friends. You don't have to become an Olympic athlete to benefit from a walking program.

Action Tips:

- Purchase a good pair of walking or cross-training shoes.

- Drink plenty of water before, during, and after your walk.

- Avoid eating a heavy meal beforehand. Stretch your calves, Achilles, thighs, back, and shoulders before and after your walk.

- Walk thirty to sixty minutes, three to five times per week.

- Walk with a friend or form a walking club. Walking partners are great motivators! If you can't walk outside, join a health club with an indoor track. Buy or rent a treadmill for your home or office.

Sixty percent of those people who have heart attacks die instantly or within an hour of the attack.

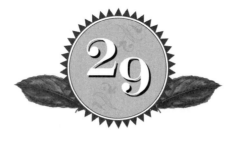

🌱

Lower Your Blood Pressure

*Learn the wisdom of compromise, for it is better to bend
a little than to break.*

—Jane Wells—

Did You Know: Almost one third of all adults in the United States have high blood pressure and half don't even know they have it. High blood pressure is a serious contender in the game of life and death, because it kills approximately thirty-three thousand Americans each year. If you have high blood pressure, your risk of having a stroke is seven times greater. More than half the people over the age of sixty-five are afflicted with hypertension or high blood pressure. African Americans in general are 20 percent more likely to have high blood pressure than whites; the risk is even higher for African Americans between the ages of twenty-four and forty-four. They are eighteen times more likely than white

Americans to experience kidney failure resulting from high blood pressure.

What's the Pressure? When you get your blood pressure level measured, it is a reading of the amount of pressure being exerted upon your blood vessel walls, particularly the arteries, as blood is pumped through your body by the heart. The top number, called systolic, is the pressure in your arteries when your heart is actively working to pump blood through your vessels. The bottom number, or the diastolic pressure, is the amount of pressure in the vessels when your heart is resting in between actual beats. Blood pressure, according to the Mayo Clinic, is normal if it is below 120/80. However there is data that indicates 115/75 millimeter Hg be the ultimate goal. And, in patients with diabetes or kidney disease, those who have blood pressure over 130/80 millimeter Hg are considered "at risk" and should consider treatment.

B.P. in Flux? Your blood pressure will "charge up" or "spike" occasionally, which is a normal response to strong emotions, stressful situations, etc. If the "spiking" occurs too frequently, it could become a risky situation.

Keep It under Wraps: Fortunately, causes of high blood pressure have been clearly defined by medical researchers. There is a wide variety of things you can do to reduce and maintain your blood pressure within a normal range.

- Cut back on sodium! Salt is a major cause of high blood pressure.

- Avoid drinking coffee if you don't indulge regularly in caffeine.

- Avoid raising your voice or shouting during an argument.

- Losing your "spare tire" if you already have high blood pressure might very well drop it to normal.

- Meditate for twenty minutes per day, consciously slowing down your breathing and heart rate.

- Avoid eating real licorice, which contains a chemical called glycyrrhizin. Glycyrrhizin causes your body to retain sodium and lose potassium.

- Eat high-potassium foods such as cantaloupe, citrus fruits, tomatoes, potatoes, and bananas.

- If you're stressed on the job, you're three times more likely to have high blood pressure.

- Walk on a treadmill and work out with weights!

- Eat more garlic, shitake mushrooms, olive oil, ocean fish, broccoli, strawberries, and green peppers. These foods all have special blood-pressure-lowering benefits. Also emphasize foods high in vitamin C and calcium.

- Stop smoking and ease up on the alcohol.

Action Tips:

- Get your blood pressure checked once a year, and more frequently if it's high.

- Before you get your blood pressure checked, arrive at least fifteen minutes early to "chill out." Leftover anxiety from getting to the doctor's office might cause a "spike" and an inaccurate reading of your blood pressure.

- Eat a diet loaded with whole grains, fresh fruits, and vegetables.

FMI:
American Heart Association, National Center,
7272 Greenville Avenue, Dallas, TX 75231
ph: 1-800-AHA-USA-1
web: www.americanheart.org

Many brands of fruit brandy, whiskey, and creme sherry contain urethane, a potent carcinogen, formed during their fermentation process!

Be a Little More Italian

Every change in the physiological state is accomplished by an appropriate change in the mental-emotional state.
—Elmer and Alice Green, Beyond Biofeedback—

Did You Know: You really need fat! Before you dive into a huge bowl of ice cream, you need to know more about essential fats. Fats are made up of smaller "pieces" of fats called fatty acids. Some are known as the "good guys," which help lower cholesterol and provide components for hormone production. While others, "the bad guys," can lead to a higher risk or cardiovascular disease and certain types of cancer. Olives, nuts, seeds, avocados, and fish are a few of the foods that provide the types of fats that we need in order to maintain optimal health. We don't need that much, but the small amount that you do obtain can lead to a variety of health benefits.

It's All Greek to Me! Researchers have been honing on the fact that the Greeks and Italians have much lower rates of cardiovascular disease and have been tying to figure out exactly what makes them tick. In a study from Italy, diets that are high in monounsaturates like olive or canola oil helped prevent unstable polyunsaturated fats from oxidizing! Polys are known not only to lower good cholesterol, but also can become oxidized and transform into artery-clogging fats. The monounsaturates provide a protective effect.

A Magic Elixir? Olive and canola oils provide essential fatty acids that cannot be synthesized in our bodies. (Cholesterol is an example of a fat we can make!) Monounsaturated fats as well as "the omegas" contain one or both of the beneficial fatty acids, linoleic or linolenic acid. Omega-3 fatty acids are found in cold-water fish, flaxseed (linseed) oil, and pumpkin. When you replace artery-clogging sat-fats, partially hydrogenated fats, and poly-fats with more healthful fats such as those that contain lineolic and/or linolenic fatty acids, you'll receive tremendous health benefits!

Out of Balance: The amount, as well as the type, of fat humans eat has changed significantly since prehistoric caveman days. Their primitive diet was likely much lower in total fat, topping out at only 21 percent of total daily calories. And only 7 to 8 percent would have been saturated fat. Hunter-gatherers' diets contained about the same amount of omega-6 and omega-3 fats, with a 1:1 ratio. Currently, most Americans eat a dietary ratio of the omegas as 20:1 and as high as 50:1

with omega-6s way out of balance. This "upside down" ratio occurred as a nation when we made an attempt to lower our saturated fats by increasing vegetable oils. Both omega-3 and omega-6 fatty acids are critical in the structure of our cell membranes and the healthy development and maintenance of our nervous system. Yet, omega-6s do not provide the health benefits that omega-3s do! Why? Omega-3s reduce inflammation and prevent excessive clotting in the blood. Too many omega-6s can increase inflammation and blood coagulation.

More Omega-3s, Please: The ideal amounts of omega-6 to omega-3 should be less than 5:1. You get plenty of omega-6s in your diet due to the high amount of vegetable oils that are used in the foods we eat on a regular basis. In order to bring your diet back into balance, taking supplements in the form of flaxseed or fish oils are your best bet! Two percent of your total daily calories should be essential fatty acids. With fast-growing bodies and brains, children need about 3 percent of their total daily intake of calories as essential fat. Preliminary research even shows depression as well as symptoms of hyperactivity and attention deficit disorder may be remedied by adding fish oils to your child's diet! And don't worry about mercury in your fish oil! Researchers at Harvard medical school found "negligible amounts of mercury" in supplements. Be sure to buy omega-3s that contain antioxidants such as vitamin E. Why? It will prevent "fish burps."

Omega-3 Benefits: It's hard to believe, but here are some of the benefits you'll receive by consuming omega-3 rich fats.

Reduced platelets sticking together in your blood, preventing blood "sludging"

Decreased blood pressure by dilating blood vessels

Activation of the immune system

Normalized blood sugar by helping insulin action

Decreased cholesterol production by your liver

Reduced inflammation

Action Tips:

- Use olive oil or canola oil tossed in a green salad or use instead of butter on bread. Add a touch of fresh garlic for extra flavor and health benefits!

- Include foods such as avocados, clarified butter, and almonds in your diet! They are all rich in monounsaturated fats!

- Buy fish oil or flaxseed oil supplements and take daily. Don't forget the antioxidants in the fish oil!

- Buy a book of food counts that provides a listing of fat grams for foods. Stick to the types of fats suggested above in order to provide optimal sources of fatty acids. Look up every food or drink you consume and keep track of those fat grams.

- Be aware that one tablespoon of olive oil contains 13.5 grams of monounsaturated fat. One whole avocado has 30 grams. But remember, it's okay because it's a good fat, as long as you cut back on bad fats (sats and polys).

- Women should limit their total dietary fat intake to a range of 20 to 40 grams, and men, 30 to 50 grams.

- Add one teaspoon of slivered almonds to your cereals or salads.

- Sauté veggies in a small amount of olive oil, or use Pam® with olive oil. Do not overheat the oil in cooking. If it smokes, it's rancid, which creates harmful peroxidases, or free radicals. If consumed too often, these might increase your risk of cancer.

- Keep your nuts and oils in the fridge to avoid rancidity. Olive oil becomes solid when chilled. To use, simply set the bottle in warm water for five minutes. Replace in your fridge when finished.

- Special Note: Avoid partially hydrogenated oils. They contain trans-fatty acids, commonly known as trans-fats. If consumed on a regular basis, trans-fats can raise "bad" cholesterol levels and create a higher risk for developing cardiovascular disease. Read labels carefully.

A wired nation? Americans consume 250 billion cups of coffee each year.

Be Your Own Nutritionist

Great souls have wills; feeble ones only have wishes.
—Chinese Proverb—

Did You Know: The only person on earth who can make a difference in your quality of life is you. Supreme beings aside, you are essentially in charge of your destiny. You know the old saying, "Where there's a will, there's a way!" Being your own nutritionist is really the only way you are going to know what is right and what is wrong for your body. If you are fortunate enough to be able to see a professional nutritionist (check out credentials—no mail-order degrees, please!) or a dietitian, it would still be helpful to have some working knowledge of your own nutritional status.

The **"Dreaded" Food Diary:** Yup! There is nothing like writing down every single morsel of food that passes your lips to give you a clear picture of your food reality. Many people are "mindless" eaters . . . they munch on something and forget about it. Then they wonder why they can't lose weight or their clothes are getting tighter. Starting today, purchase a small notebook and list in the columns at the top of each page: Type of Food, Amount (ounces, tablespoons, cups, etc.), Time of Day, Place, and General Feelings. Keep track of what you eat for seven days. Then, using a book of food counts, calculate the number of calories, grams of protein, grams of fat, and grams of carbohydrates and create totals per day. The following are what you need to look for:

	Women	Men
Calories	1,200 to 2,200	1,800 to 2,800
Fat	20 to 40 grams	30 to 50 grams
Protein	40 to 60 grams	50 to 80 grams

**Pregnant women need up to one hundred grams of protein daily.
**Endurance athletes need the most protein. (See "Keep Protein in Perspective")

These amounts are equivalent to between six and eleven servings of carbs per day, with one slice of whole-grain bread or one small potato representing one serving each.

If you find your numbers do not fall in these ranges, your nutritional profile is out of balance. You need to put it back in balance. Be sure you eat frequently throughout the day, get plenty of complex carbohydrates, a small amount of lean protein, and a bit of essential fat in your diet daily. Iced tea, soft drinks, coffee, and hot tea are poor substitutes for clear water. Stay away from fast or frozen foods. Avoid those drive-through windows! Try to focus on fresh foods.

You are unique! Some of us need more protein than others. Some need a little more essential fat; others do better on predominately a high carbohydrate or "semi-vegetarian" diet (see "Be a Semi-Vegetarian"). But most of all, focus on how you feel physically.

Can't Change Your Matter if You Don't Change Your Mind: Consider keeping a food diary as a reintroduction to yourself. Try to look objectively at what you eat, removing words such as *bad* and *terrible* from your dietary assessment. Accept yourself as simply human. Meditate on what it will feel like to be at your goal weight. Don't dwell upon how difficult the process will be. Tell yourself that you deserve to weigh what you want to weigh, and really feel it! Don't be impatient. Proceed as if you were an objective observer in the process. Under the "General Feelings" column in your diary, observe how connected you are emotionally with your eating experience. Do you eat when stressed? Depressed? If so, find other outlets for those negative feelings and try to eat when your stomach wants food, not your heart or your mind.

Remember the Tortoise and the Hare? Studies have shown that people who lose weight or body fat at a rate not exceeding two pounds per week will be more likely to keep the weight off in the end. Liquid diets, starvation programs (less than twelve hundred calories per day), and the use of diet pills do not keep the weight off! As a matter of fact, more than 90 percent of people who lose weight on these types of programs gain the weight back. Just think of all the money you are spending and the cash the diet companies are making! They feed like sharks upon your failures! Being your own nutritionist will hopefully prevent you from falling prey to these parasitic programs! And lastly, changing your behavior along with gradual weight loss while on a sensible eating plan are some keys to success.

Action Tip:

- Keep a food diary for at least seven days. Continue to maintain a food record while you are in the process of changing your eating habits. Keep track of every morsel of food, beverages, and bits of gums and candy that go into your mouth. Count everything! Keep a positive, objective attitude!

•

FMI:
Review the following chapters in this book:
"Make Picasso Proud," "Get a Handle on Those 'Sat-Fats," "Tap into Clean Water," "Get Energized with Carbohydrates," "Become a Semi-vegetarian," and "Keep Protein in Perspective."

Only 4 percent of Americans are satisfied with their physical appearance.

Save Your Skin

*Age is not a handicap. Age is nothing but a number.
It is how you use it.*

—Ethel Payne—

Did You Know: As you age, your skin cells naturally slow down in the production of collagen, which is essential for maintaining the integrity of your skin's flexible structure. Toxicants such as smoke, air pollution, and foreign chemicals in the water and food you consume can have a negative impact upon the appearance of your skin. Your skin is highly receptive to how well nourished you are, how much you do or don't exercise, stress, and sun exposure. Experts have found that all you have to do is follow a few "skin healthy" rules and you won't have to be a victim of the aging process.

The Skinny on Skin: Your skin is primarily made up of two layers, the epidermis (or outer layer) and the dermis (lower layer). The epidermis is actually comprised of two parts, with the top part being made up of dead, flattened, keratinized cells. These dead cells originate from living cells that have moved up from the basal layer of the epidermis. Once the dead cells have moved to the surface, they are naturally sloughed off through bathing, rubbing on your clothing, or by simply drying out and falling off! The lower layer or dermis of your skin is much thicker than the epidermis and contains blood cells, nerves, sweat glands, and hair follicles and is also the place where new skin cells and collagen production originate. People with an optimal diet, who have minimal exposure to enemies of the skin, are much more likely to have a more youthful epidermis. New cell growth and reproduction are highly dependent upon these two factors.

Enemies of the Epidermis! Aging, wrinkling, and skin cancer can all be a result of not only damage from the outside in but also from the inside out. When cell membranes are damaged, they respond accordingly by getting a little thicker than before, such as in scarring from an actual wound. The skin cells, even at the deepest layer of the basal tissue, might become damaged from smoking or breathing in polluted air. Your external layers of cells typically protect themselves from sun damage by creating pigment. The more pigment a skin contains; the less likely the cells will be susceptible to damage. African-Americans are less likely to experience sunburn, sun-induced wrinkling, and even skin cancer, due to the high levels of pigmentation. The fairer your skin, the lighter your eyes and hair, the more susceptible you will be to the ravages of aging and skin damage. Skin-damaging free radicals are created in your body when you smoke, live, and/or work in a large, polluted city; consume foods or beverages that contain significant amounts of questionable chemicals; and when you spend a lot of time in the sun. These free radicals damage new skin cell membranes, creating tougher, rigid cells, which contribute to the formation of wrinkles! Other wrinkle factors include excessive stress, a bad attitude, continuous frowning, and lack of exercise, which is needed to bring oxygen to developing cells.

Skin Friends: Eating a diet high in the A. C. E. team (antioxidant vitamins A, C, and E) and other antioxidants, can definitely contribute to the "youth factor" many of us are seeking! If you regularly load up on foods rich in antioxidants, especially "the powerful three," you'll also lessen your risk of getting skin cancer, or melanoma. Drinking plenty of purified bottled water not containing fluoride (fluoride might damage dermis cells) will keep your skin properly hydrated. Eating small amounts of food high in essential fatty acids such as avocados, nuts, nut butter, seeds, olives, olive oil, canola oil, salmon, halibut, etc. will provide the right components for optimal skin cell production.

Beta Skin: If you eat foods containing beta-carotene—such as carrots, cantaloupe, sweet potatoes, and apricots—you can acquire a protective effect due to your skin getting a "tan"

from carotene buildup in your skin cells. Sun-sensitive individuals who had increased their beta-carotene intake over a period of four to six weeks found they could increase their time in the sun by up to 84 percent longer in one study. Some were given up to 50 milligrams of beta-carotene, 300 percent over the present RDA, without any toxic side effects.

"C" the Light: Vitamin C also has natural sunscreen qualities that protect your skin. Dr. Sheldon Pinnell of Duke University Medical Center, found that when he applied a topical vitamin C solution to the skin of pigs, they were able to withstand ultraviolet light exposure up to five times the normal time it would take to give them sunburn. Topical vitamin C protects the skin by screening out harmful rays, while allowing vitamin D synthesis to occur. Commercial sunscreens block vitamin D synthesis. The topical vitamin C sunscreen effects lasted for *three* days, even after the pigs were scrubbed down several times! This particular formula is not commercially available. One other great benefits of the topical vitamin C is that it appears not only to prevent skin damage and premature aging, but it also might stimulate collagen synthesis, which is of ultimate importance in maintaining the integrity of your skin. Foods high in bioflavanoids work right alongside vitamin C in keeping skin healthy. Tomatoes, apricots, broccoli, grapes, cantaloupe, cherries, and the pulp of citrus fruits (not orange or grapefruit) are excellent sources of bioflavanoids.

Skin Tricks: According to a study in the *British Journal of Dermatology,* people who scrubbed their skin daily with a lightly abrasive skin cleanser (Brasivol) caused their epidermis to become thicker and more youthful. The topical drug Retin A has a similar effect when applied to the skin. Scrubbing might be cheaper! Hyaluronic acid derived from fruits such as apples or grapes and products containing mucopolysaccharides, such as pure aloe vera gel, have also been found to have some skin benefits.

Keep It Healthy! Sun damage is the number-one factor in the development of skin cancer. Applying a sunscreen that protects against both UVA and UVB rays thirty to forty-five minutes before sun exposure will provide an optimal shield from harmful rays. The SPF factor tells you the length of time you can spend in the sun without burning. For example, SPF 15 means you can spend fifteen times longer than if you used no sunscreen. Be sure to reapply frequently if you swim or sweat quite a bit. Look for the seal of approval from the Skin Cancer Foundation on the label. If you're on medication, check with your doctor before you go out in the sun, because some medications make your skin more sensitive.

Action Tips:

- Eat plenty of foods high in beta-carotene and vitamin C. Examples are carrots, pumpkin, sweet potatoes, spinach, cantaloupe, greens, kale, Swiss chard, butternut squash, mangoes, tomato-vegetable juice, strawberries, kiwis, red and green peppers, oranges, grapefruit, papayas, strawberries, kiwis, red and green peppers, broccoli, Brussels sprouts, grapefruit, cauliflower, and kale.

- Seek out skin creams that contain vitamin C and/or other fruit acids or mucopolysaccharides.

- If you smoke or are exposed to secondhand smoke or city pollution on a regular basis, double up on antioxidant-rich foods.

- Always use a sunscreen when sun exposure is inevitable!

According to the Center for Disease Control in Atlanta, the couch potato lifestyle is responsible for two hundred thousand preventable deaths each year.

Cut the Fat with Ten Quick Tips

It has long been an axiom of mine that the little things are infinitely more important.

—Sir Arthur Conan Doyle—

Here Goes . . . the Fastest Fat Tips: These tips will help you lower cholesterol, lose body fat, and decrease your risk of cancer, heart attack, and stroke.

1. If you love eggs, you need to know that they have a whopping 45 calories or 5 grams of saturated fat! You can cut those grams out by substituting two egg whites and one-quarter cup of an egg substitute. Prepare scrambled eggs, omelets, and baking recipes with this mixture.

2. If you're a milk lover and you can't seem to nudge yourself or your family to go lower than 2 percent, try mixing in half skim milk and gradually increase the ratio each week until the carton is almost all skim.

3. When sautéing your favorite veggies or lean meat, use an olive-oil-based spray such as *Pam*. Not only will you reduce the amount of fat calories consumed, but you'll get a small amount of the good kind of fat, monounsaturated fat, which has been shown to decrease low-density lipoprotein cholesterol—the bad kind.

4. Do you like ground beef? Even lean ground beef packs a heavy "fat wallop" upon your body. Try substituting ground chicken or turkey breast in tacos, spaghetti sauces, and meat loaf.

5. If a recipe calls for using oil, such as in many muffin recipes, use the equivalent amount of applesauce to produce your own tasty and moist, low-fat versions.

6. Use fat-free sour cream, cream cheese, and cottage cheese as great alternatives to their fat-laden cousins! For melting, mix fat-free cheeses with low-fat types to obtain a more genuine, cheesy texture and flavor.

7. Choose healthy cookie alternatives that are trans-fat free. Check out whole food-oriented markets where you'll find a wide variety of delicious low-fat, whole-grain cookies, muffins, and granola. Fig bars, graham crackers, vanilla wafers, ginger snaps, and animal crackers are all healthy, low-fat alternatives.

8. When ordering in a restaurant, be sure to hone in on the items on the menu that are grilled, broiled, or steamed. As a comparison, one five-ounce piece of fried fish could

pack a walloping 18 to 20 grams of fat. If the fish were grilled, it would contain only 3 grams of total fat. Also ask for veggies to be prepared without any oil or fat!

9. When counting fat grams, don't tell the entire world about it, or the diet saboteurs will be coming out of the woodwork! You know the type. If you look the other way, they'll slip a pat of butter in your potatoes! Those "grannies" will do it every time! The bottom line is you need to be subtle about your transition and commitment to better health. And one last trick: if you are in a situation where others are imposing a sumptuous dessert upon you, fake it and say your stomach isn't feeling that wonderful and ask if you can take a rain check. Hey, it's a great survival technique!

FMI:
Cooking Light magazine, P.O. Box 62376, Tampa, FL 33662
(800) 336-0125 www.cookinglight.com

Eating salty foods when you are under stress can make you feel even more stressed out.

Chill Out with Calcium

We should pray for a sane mind in a sound body.

—Juvenal—

Did You Know: You probably aren't getting enough calcium in your daily diet, just like many other typical Americans. Obtaining adequate amounts is absolutely essential to acquiring and maintaining a strong, healthy, lean body; a calm nervous system; and a clear head! Here are a few reasons why you need to make an effort to eat foods high in this mineral every day:

- Your body contains about two and a half pounds of calcium, with 99 percent present in your bones and teeth, and 1 percent floating around in your bloodstream and in cellular fluids. You need enough calcium to maintain these optimal levels.

- Six to seven hundred milligrams of calcium are being used up every day in the new growth and repair of your bones.

- Calcium helps activate specific enzymes to break down fats and proteins.

- Calcium is essential to clotting in your blood.

- Calcium assists in the transmission of messages throughout your nervous system.

- Calcium regulates contraction and relaxation of muscles, including your heart muscle.

- Calcium aids in the absorption of a wide variety of nutrients.

- Women over the age of fifty, due to a drop in estrogen levels, are at high risk of developing osteoporosis. Calcium supplements are recommended at a maximum level of 1,500 milligrams.

- The RDA for calcium for healthy men is 1,000 milligrams to 1,300 milligrams; for women 1,000 to 1,200 milligrams; 1,300 milligrams for teens; and 1,200 milligrams for pregnant and lactating women as well as for adults over the age of fifty. Two-thirds of the women in the United States are not getting the RDA! Guys get closer to the required amount because of how many more nutrient-rich calories they can eat as compared to their female counterparts!

Burn Body Fat Faster! The team at the Nutrition Institute at the University of Tennessee at Knoxville have concluded a diet high in calcium can enhance how well your body burns fat. Mice given more calcium than others burned up to 69 percent more body fat than those who did not have high calcium in their diets. Calcium appears to increase thermogenesis, indicated by increase in body core temperature. Researchers found when there was more calcium in the cell, more fat was burned. Sources of calcium given to the mice ranged from calcium supplements to medium and high doses of nonfat dry milk. Those who had the most calcium burned up the most fat! Be sure when you begin to add more calcium to your diet you choose low-fat or nonfat sources. Choose nonfat and low-fat sources of calcium, especially when adding dairy. Dairy can add a big "saturated fat" punch if you don't watch out.

On the Horizon: Many studies are constantly being conducted on the health benefits of calcium, the latest findings being directly related to controlling blood pressure. In one study, women were given a 1,500 milligram calcium supplement and found it to be directly related to a drop in high blood pressure levels. Other studies show a relationship between lower rates of colon cancer and adequate dietary calcium intake.

Get Your Calcium Here! Dairy products such as yogurt, acidophilus, regular milk, and low-fat cheeses are excellent sources of calcium. But many people can't tolerate them due to lactose or milk sugar intolerance or milk protein allergies.

Canned salmon and sardines, collard greens, mustard and turnip greens, broccoli, kale, soybeans, tofu, almonds, oysters, clams, and shrimp are all excellent non-dairy alternatives for obtaining adequate amounts of calcium.

The Big Blockers: Certain foods and beverages will block the absorption of calcium into your bloodstream. They are alcohol, spinach, parsley, beet greens, rhubarb, excessive fiber, soft drinks with phosphoric acid (no citric acid), caffeine, salt, bran, and oatmeal. Just don't include these foods or beverages along with your high-calcium meal. Wait an hour after your morning cup of coffee to have your yogurt mixed with a few slivered almonds!

Action Tips:

- Keep track of how much calcium you have in an entire day. Be sure to count non-dairy sources.

- Make an effort to obtain calcium every day from other sources besides milk products.

- Take a calcium supplement.

Tofu has two cancer-fighting chemicals, genistein and daidzein, which inhibit the growth of tumors by cutting off their developing blood supply. One quarter of a tofu block daily will do!

Get a Little Culture

Men take more pains to mask than mend.
—Benjamin Franklin—

Good for You, Bacteria! Lactobacillus Acidophilus. What's that, you say? It's the good bacteria also known as a member of the family of probiotics. Probiotics are various strains of "good" bacteria found in healthy large intestines. This good bacteria is needed for proper breakdown and absorption of nutrients. A higher level of friendly bacteria in the intestines prevents the invasion of bad bacteria or pathogens from colonizing! Friendly bacteria, such as acidophilus and bifidus, aid the immune system and digestion and synthesize vitamins in the intestine. Candida albicans, natural yeast found in the body, can grow rapidly if the "good guy/bad guy" bacterial balance is out of whack! This yeast can promote infection if it is allowed to get out of hand.

Halitosis? Bad breath, if not dentally or orally related, can often be taken care of by supplementing with acidophilus or eating yogurt made with it. Drink acidophilus milk—it's easy to find. It's sometimes difficult to find yogurt with acidophilus by itself—and if the cultures have been added before the heating process (pasteurization), the live bacteria is killed. We need the living stuff! The best kind is named Bulgarian yogurt. It has a zesty flavor, nothing like highly processed varieties, yet it contains a healthy amount of living or good bacteria.

Yeastie Beasties: Studies at Long Island Jewish Medical Center in New York found that women eating yogurt cultures with lactobacillus acidophilus experienced significantly lower occurrences of yeast infections.

What's a Healthy Colon? In order to clinically assess the health of your large intestine you can request a lab count of the ratio of your good bacteria such as lactobacillus acidophilus to the unfriendly types! According to Dr. James Balch, MD, and Phyllis Balch, CNC, coauthors of *Prescription for Nutritional Healing,* a ratio of 85 percent to 15 percent is desirable. If you are one of those people who experience frequent bloating and constipation, an acidophilus "look see" is in order. If you find you're out of balance, you can fix it and feel better!

The Fix-It Stuff! Just by drinking milk containing acidophilus or cultured milk beverages such as kefir and other yogurt drinks, you will probably help reestablish bacterial balance.

Eating yogurt containing live "good bacteria" cultures may help reduce yeast infections. If the dairy methods don't turn you on or you're sensitive to milk (as many people are), taking a probiotic supplement is a good alternative. One to two capsules with each meal is recommended and will provide the following benefits:

- Aids digestion

- Relieves diarrhea and constipation

- Helps colitis and diverticulitis

- Enhances nutrient absorption

- Fights bad breath from stagnant colon

- Clears up skin disorders

- Assists in the combat against certain bad bacteria and illnesses

Research has shown how probiotics can be used to treat diarrhea and constipation. One study revealed that forty-five of forty-nine constipation sufferers found relief, while sixteen of seventeen diarrhea patients were helped significantly by taking a probiotic supplement.

The Ultimate Travel Aid: Savvy travelers have caught on to the idea of probiotic "loading" two weeks before taking a trip to another country, especially those where Montezuma's revenge is common. It turns out that increasing the amount of probiotics helps prevent the bad bacteria from making you ill.

A Cancer Fighter? Yup! When probiotics were given to volunteers for an entire month, it was found that there was a significant decline in the types of enzymes that normally turn other things into cancer-causing agents.

Candida—the Controversy. William Crook, MD, published a book in 1983 called *The Yeast Connection*. It proposed that if the yeastie beasties get out of control they might spread into the body, causing a release of a toxin that might make one feel fatigued, depressed, headachy, and sore and cause pains and digestive problems. The proposed treatment is to eat a diet that will starve the yeasts. Therefore, any sugar, alcohol, aged cheese, or other foods containing yeast should be eliminated. The conventional medical community has balked at this theory because it is lacking scientific evidence to support it. However, most doctors admit the diet would help almost everyone feel better, regardless of their condition, but they have a problem with some of the pharmaceutical drugs recommended.

Action Tips:

- Include probiotics in your life. Small children and infants, if not breast-fed, would benefit from the consumption of some form of probiotics.

- Eat foods containing "good" bacteria. Cultured yogurt (goat's milk or soy yogurt are available if you are sensitive to cow's milk), buttermilk, kefir, and acidophilus milk are excellent sources.

- Take a probiotic supplement per instructions on the label. (Warning: If you have high levels of yeast you might experience bloating when probiotics are first introduced as a supplement. This will eventually be alleviated.)

- Get a count of the ratio of good bacteria in your system—85 percent to 15 percent is a good ratio.

Apples are a member of the rose family.

Preserve Thyself with the Relaxation Response

Learn how to relax . . . for fast-acting relief— try slowing down!

—Lily Tomlin—

Did You Know: Nine out of ten Americans say they experience some form of stress one to two times per week, and one in four estimates stress happens every day. According to a study by the American Institute of Stress, 75 percent to 90 percent of all doctor visits are somehow related to stress! There are those that seem to let things slide right off of their backs, while others might get tense if a line in a grocery store is moving a little too slowly. This is the big difference.

The Natural Nemesis: Feelings of anxiety, tension, and stress have their roots in the beginning of mankind. If early man was faced with a life-threatening situation, these feelings

189

would allow him to get the heck out of there! If these feelings did not exist, well, maybe man wouldn't have survived. The problem is modern man has these primitive stress responses in a modern society that doesn't accommodate a natural reaction or release of these feelings. The analogy of feeling bottled up is so appropriate for many! Some people deal with stress productively, using exercise, creative outlets, or just plain zoning out as tools. Others might constantly experience the highs and lows of emotions such as anger and fear. When these feelings are experienced, blood pressure is elevated. This elevation is the number one cause of heart attacks and stroke. Stress can also weaken your immune systems. Relaxation techniques help you to have more energy, increase your alertness, and make you less likely to use destructive means of stress release such as drugs, alcohol, and other debilitating behaviors.

Preserve Thyself! If you value your life, friends and family included, self-preservation is a must—especially for those who experience violent, primitive feelings more often than others. Stress unchecked will make you sick. Herbert Benson, MD, author of *The Relaxation Response,* claims that utilizing a relaxation technique only ten to twenty minutes two times per day can greatly improve our quality of life. Here's what he says are the four components necessary to any relaxation program:

- A quiet environment

- Focusing on an object or symbol or a specific feeling

- A positive attitude (leave your type-A feelings outside)

- Finding a comfortable position (sitting as opposed to lying down—you might fall asleep!)

Action Tips:

- Create a quiet environment to meditate in twice a day for about fifteen minutes per session.

- Sit quietly with your legs closed and feet flat on the floor, hands resting comfortably.

- Focus on relaxing every muscle group, beginning with the toes and moving throughout your body.

- Keep your mouth closed and breathe in through your nose. Exhale through your mouth, relaxing with every movement.

- Relax for ten to twenty minutes, but when you have completed your session sit quietly and get comfortable with your alertness level before getting up.

- During the entire process, it is important not to get uptight if other thoughts are drifting in and out. Eventually, you can train yourself to relax, completely focusing on your object or feelings.

- Make sure you set aside the time to do these exercises daily.

FMI:
The American Institute of Stress, 124 Park Avenue, Yonkers, NY 10703
ph: 914 963-1200 web: www.stress.org

The Benson-Henry Institute for Mind Body Medicine,
824 Boylston Street, Chestnut Hill, MA 02467
ph: 617-732-9130 web: www.mbmi.org

The Relaxation Response, Herbert Benson, MD,
Avon Books, New York, 1985

Americans are eating 557 percent more broccoli today than they did in 1971.

Unwind with Endorphins

You cannot have a future unless you think about the future.
—John Galsworthy—

Did You Know: People who exercise regularly are better able to deal with stress than those who don't. People who exercise aerobically recover from a stressful event faster. A fit person during a stress test on a treadmill will experience a quicker return to normal heart rate and blood pressure than a more sedentary person of the same weight. A healthy person's arteries are flexible and open up during stress. On the other hand, a person with cardiovascular disease has constricted or inflexible arteries that keep his heart rate and blood pressure high after stress. Research shows people who exercise on a daily basis can handle stress more readily than a person who does not exercise. Known as a mood booster, exercise has also been shown to alleviate anxiety and depression.

Details, Please: Your body has the ability to produce natural opiates or morphine-like chemicals. When they are released in the brain, they inhibit cells that deal with pain, behavior, pleasure, and emotions! During exercise your pituitary gland releases more of one of these agents called beta endorphin. The exercise high has been traced to more of this chemical traveling through your bloodstream. Exercisers often refer to it as a euphoric feeling. So, exercising aerobically not only benefits your heart and lung system, it gives your brain a workout, too! The blood flow to your brain increases up to one-third more than at resting states. Exercise can also stimulate creativity by creating an alpha or relaxing state in your brain-wave activity. Thus, creative blocks can be destroyed simply by taking a thirty-minute spin on your bike! So you see, unwinding with endorphins released through exercise can enhance many areas of your life!

A Natural Pain Reliever: Your body has its own pain-killing system or analgesic system that blocks pain signals before they reach the brain. Endorphins are a central part of this pain-relieving system since they are secreted into the bloodstream during times of pain or stress. How do they work? Endorphins prevent neurotransmitters from sending pain signals to the nerves. Ever notice that once you start exercising your pains suddenly diminish? In one study, athletes' pain thresholds were measured. It was found their pain tolerance, during intense exercise, increased a whopping 53 percent as compared to when they were not exercising.

A Few More Endorphin Facts:

- People who are wound up tight were found to have less electrical activity or sparks that cause tension in their muscles following a workout.

- The average result of an exercise session is a euphoric or endorphin high for up to two hours per workout.

Action Tips:

- If you have moderate stress in your life (and who doesn't?) exercising aerobically thirty to sixty minutes three to four times per week will be a great benefit to you.

- For those who consider themselves high-stress victims, exercising for twenty minutes six to seven times per week might do the trick.

- Practicing yoga or similar movements (you can even get a home video to follow) has also been shown to open the door to release endorphins.

- Acupuncture increases the amount of endorphins pro-duced during the after treatment—and you don't even have to move! Now you couch potatoes have no excuse for not unlocking your endorphins to help you on your way to a longer, healthier life!

The average American opens his or her refrigerator twenty-two times a day.

Ease on Down the Road with "E"

Without knowledge, life is not more than the shadow of death.

—Molière—

Did You Know: People with heart pain known as angina, elderly individuals who lose some of their mental reasoning abilities, and those with cataracts have one thing in common—lower than normal amounts of vitamin E in their bloodstreams! Many researchers have turned their attention to this powerful antioxidant, the third member of the A. C. E. team (together with vitamins A and C). Vitamin E keeps your body healthy by preventing the breakdown of certain cells that could potentially turn into damaging free radicals. When a cell, such as a lipid, or fat, is floating around and becomes unstable, it might pick up an oxygen molecule. This process forms a "free radical." A little oxygen can't hurt, right? Wrong!

Once oxygen enters the picture, a free radical is formed that potentially could be very harmful to your health, possibly contributing to heart disease or cancer. Vitamin E, an antioxidant, protects cells from picking up that extra oxygen, hence allowing the cells to remain in a more healthy state.

Histor-E Lesson: Discovered in 1922, vitamin E is not a single compound, but rather an entire family of compounds with eight structurally related forms, or isomers. The eight isomers are made up of four tocopherols (alpha, beta, gamma, and delta tocopherol) and four tocotrienols, also known by their alpha, beta, gamma, and delta forms. While all forms of vitamin E are potent membrane-soluble antioxidants, only two—alpha tocopherol and gamma tocopherol—are the most commonly found in nature.

"E" Basics: Vitamin E is a fat soluble and is absorbed in your large intestines, where fat absorption occurs as well. Because it is fat soluble, it is readily absorbed and stored in a variety of places in your body, including your fat tissues, liver, heart, blood, uterus, testes, and adrenal and pituitary glands. However, it doesn't stay stored for very long, so you need to eat foods that are rich in vitamin E on a fairly regular basis and/or take a supplement. A combination of gamma and alpha-tocopherol is the best source of vitamin E. While the alpha tocopherol form of vitamin E has long been valued as a potent antioxidant, its little-known cousin, gamma tocopherol, may be equally important in promoting health and protecting against disease. Found in nuts, seeds, and vegetable oils, gamma tocopherol accounts for about 70 percent of the vitamin E in the North American diet. The Recommended Daily Allowance or RDA for a healthy adult, nineteen years of age or older is 15 milligrams or 22.5 International Units (IU).

More Details: Many researchers believe that clogging of the arteries occurs due to fats being oxidized in your bloodstream. After they go through this transformation, they are very likely to settle down right there on the interior walls of your arteries and blood vessels. The buildup continues as more and more fats break down into lipid peroxidases (broken down fats with oxygen along for the ride), which in turn might cause narrowing or blockages to occur. Heart attacks and strokes are often the direct result of this type of buildup. Antioxidant E plays a key preventative role in this scenario.

The Amazing E: The World Health Organization announced in January 1991 that the level of vitamin E in our bloodstreams was a better predictor of death than were risk factors such as smoking, high blood pressure, and high cholesterol.

Cataracts in elderly people go hand in hand with vitamin E deficiency. The theory is senile cataracts might be caused by free radical damage to the eye. Vitamin E supplementation in the elderly prevents the development of cataracts. In addition, animal studies in India showed that clouding of the cornea or the transparent covering of the eye was directly related to vitamin E deficiency.

Jeffrey Blumberg, PhD, found that men who exercised and took a vitamin E supplement experienced less damage to muscle and connective tissues than those who didn't take E.

Joel Schwartz, DMD, found the combination of vitamins A and E killed cancer cells in test tubes. In other studies looking at the combination of vitamins E and A, there appears to be a synergistic effect between the nutrients in the prevention of the growth of cancers.

There are many other studies that associate vitamin E supplementation and improvement and health in a wide variety of areas, including boosting the immune system and increased resistance to bacterial infection, alleviating painful fibrocystic breast conditions, improving the health of gums, alleviating PMS symptoms, and avoiding lung tissue damage from ozone and air pollution inhalation. (People who exercise outdoors in polluted areas would benefit from taking vitamin E, since pollution is a major cause of free-radical formation in the body.)

Action Tips:

- Eat foods high in vitamin E. These include cold-pressed vegetable oils, Brussels sprouts, leafy greens, wheat germ, nuts, seeds, and legumes.

- If you want to take a vitamin E supplement, do not take it at the same time as an iron supplement, because the iron will use up the E! Take them eight hours apart. The intake of four hundred IUs per day appears to be beneficial to preventing the development of heart disease and cancer.

- If you exercise you need more vitamin E than those who are less active.

- Our needs for vitamin E go up with age. Either eat more wheat germ or consider taking a supplement!

- If you are taking fish oil supplements or eat quite a bit of fatty fish or unsaturated fats, your need for vitamin E goes up.

- Most vitamin E capsules are oil-based. If you have a diagnosed condition where fat absorption is a problem, consider taking the dry-form supplement because it will be more easily absorbed.

The average human heart beats about one hundred thousand times every twenty-four hours.

Be a Semi-Vegetarian

The greater part of our happiness or misery depends on our dispositions and not on our circumstances.

—Martha Washington—

Did You Know: Want to live to one hundred years old? The people from the Japanese island of Okinawa appear to have found the answer. On this small island, there are four hundred twenty-seven people over the age of one hundred, in a population of just 1.27 million. That's nearly four times the average number of the West. Rates of heart disease, cancer, and stroke are the lowest in the world, and the menopause occurs ten years later than in the West. So how do they do it? A high level of soy, vegetables, fish, and low levels of alcohol play a part, as does a high level of physical activity well into old age. Stress is also low. They consume 30 percent or less of their diet as fat and keep salt intake low. With recommendations from the American Cancer Institute, American Heart Association, and the United States Department of Agriculture (USDA) to cut back on saturated fats and cholesterol, it has become a natural transition to move in the direction of eating less animal protein and more of the vegetarian protein sources. Because most of our commercial meat and meat products contain cholesterol-raising fats, eating more like a vegetarian might make you healthier! A mere 4 ounces of white meat chicken without the skin contains 5 grams of saturated fat and 96 milligrams of cholesterol. The American Heart Association recommends a maximum of 300 milligrams daily for healthy individuals and 100 milligrams for those with elevated cholesterol!

Be a Part-Timer! Excess consumption of red meat increases the risk of heart disease, certain cancers, and other disorders. As a result, health-conscious people are eating more fruit, vegetables, and fish and are staying away from beef. With all the benefits attributed to plant foods, it appears vegetarians enjoy a huge life-span advantage over meat eaters! Eating one or two meals per day as a vegetarian and saving one meal, preferably lunch, as your protein meal will have a positive impact upon your health, energy, and level of stress. Your digestive tract will welcome the abundance of fiber-rich grains, legumes, fruits, and vegetables. Loaded with plenty of high-energy carbohydrates, cholesterol-lowering soluble and insoluble fibers, and plenty of antioxidant-rich nutrients, you'll be giving your body a tremendous health boost! Animal proteins simply do not contain any fiber whatsoever! As a matter of fact, they can easily stay in your digestive tract for a period of three days if you abstain from eating high-fiber foods along with them!

The How-To's:

- If you haven't done so, gradually begin to add more whole grains and fresh produce to your diet.

- Begin to decrease the amount of meat or chicken you eat at your main meal. If you can't cut back during dinner, then do so at lunch. Your goal is to have no more than six ounces total per day.

- Begin to focus on vegetarian types of entrees such as black beans and brown rice, pinto beans and soft corn tortillas, pasta and spaghetti sauce with mushrooms, and other veggies.

- Try to include a tossed green salad and/or fresh fruit during lunch and dinner.

- Snack on apples, pears, citrus fruits, rice cakes, baked tortilla chips, mashed pinto beans, etc.

- Be sure to drink plenty of water to accommodate your new eating style.

- Eat a breakfast based on whole grains such as high-fiber cereals, whole-grain pancakes or waffles, and some fruit.

- If you want to improve your quality of sleep, eat your protein at lunch. Carbohydrates without protein help induce a relaxed state by allowing your brain to produce more serotonin, a calming brain chemical.

- Stock up on a few good vegetarian cookbooks and experiment!

Why Not Go Total Vegetarian? Vegetarians do benefit from the antioxidants, anticarcinogens, and fiber found naturally in plant sources. However, many physicians do not recommend vegetarian diets for reversing heart disease and various other disease states. It turns out that one in ten experience stomach and intestinal problems and lower energy on a complete vegetarian diet. Nutritionists who specialize in vegetarianism find that if not properly executed, a vegetarian diet can have deleterious effects. People may trade health problems associated with excess for those that originate in scarcity. Dr. Weston Price, a pioneer in the study of dietary patterns in primitive cultures, traveled all over the world and observed the diets of traditional cultures where dental caries, or cavities, and degenerative diseases didn't exist. After twenty years of searching, Dr. Price claimed he did not find one of these cultures that did not eat some form of animal products. The healthiest cultures included seafood and/or wild game and grass-fed animals in their diets. These forms of animal protein contain high amounts of EPA, an essential fatty acid known to have cholesterol and blood pressure-lowering qualities.

.

A Veggie Recommendation: If you have high cholesterol and/or blood pressure, heart disease, diabetes, or any other disease condition known to respond positively to dietary and lifestyle changes, go ahead and check out a balanced vegetarian-oriented program. Once your health improves, don't feel guilty about becoming a "semi-vegetarian."

Action Tips:

- Begin slowly and maintain optimism.

- Try it with a friend or spouse.

- Take a vegetarian cooking class.

FMI:
www.vegetariantimes.com

Sixteen million Americans suffer from ulcers.

Slow Down on the Sugar

Clogged with yesterday's excess, the body drags the mind down with it.

—Horace—

Did You Know: Although traditional recommendations suggest a diet with 65 percent of calories supplied by complex carbohydrates, high-carbohydrate diets still increase blood sugar and stimulate insulin production. The key is to eat a balanced diet of complex carbohydrates along with moderate protein and essential fat sources. Carbohydrates will raise your blood sugar. The key is to eat high fiber carbs that ultimately release glucose into your system slowly. High fiber carbs are thought to have a high glycemic load. The glycemic index rates foods on how much they raise your blood sugar. The less of an impact upon your blood sugar at one time, the healthier typically the food is as an energy source. Eating too many sugary foods might calm you down, but also give you an adrenaline rush, destroy vital minerals and vitamins, slow down your digestion, and decay your teeth! According to the latest food pyramid recommendation by the United States Department of Agriculture (USDA), you should not consume more than 10 percent of your total daily calories from processed sugary foods. Unfortunately, when it comes to eating sweet treats our intellect is not necessarily dictating our rationale!

First Love: Let's face it; humans love sugar. Newborn infants who receive sugar water during their first days of life appear to have a higher tolerance to uncomfortable procedures, such as circumcisions. The babies seem much calmer than their counterpart's not drinking sugar. This is not to say that drinking sugar water is the most healthful thing for a newborn to drink. We are attracted to the wonderful pleasurable sweetness of sugary-tasting foods. Some researchers believe our attraction to sweet-tasting food originates to the days when just surviving was the name of the game. Sweet-tasting foods were safe, and bitter foods were typically poisonous. Sugary foods can make us feel calmer, as illustrated with newborn babies. Our brains respond to eating sugar by releasing serotonin, a brain chemical that makes us feel calm and happy.

Sweet Addiction: Did you ever notice that when you are depressed or sad, you don't want a steak. You want ice cream or sweets. Scientists speculate that brain chemicals, which are altered by antidepressant drugs, are also affected by the foods we eat. For example, many people, including those who are depressed, are sugar-sensitive. Eating sweets gives them a temporary emotional boost, which leads to a craving for still more sweets. Some researchers believe sugar may be addictive! Researchers studied rats induced to binge on sugar and found that they showed telltale signs of withdrawal, including the shakes and changes in brain chemistry, when the effects of the sweets were blocked. These signs are similar to those produced by drug withdrawal.

Sugar, Not Just Bad for Your Teeth: Sugar may be bad for your blood vessels and many other areas of the body. In a study of fourteen healthy men and women who drank the equivalent of two cans of soda, the results showed excess sugar in the bloodstream stimulated the formation of free radicals. This may explain the association between high sugar diets and plaque build up due to how free radicals can cause damage to blood vessels. When damage occurs, blockage of arteries and cardiovascular disease may be the result.

Sugar As Energy: Carbohydrates are the main nutrient in our diets that provide us with energy. Simple carbohydrates provide the quickest source of energy to your body, which, when metabolized, release glucose very quickly into your bloodstream. Complex carbohydrates take longer to break down, releasing energy or glucose molecules more slowly. Whereas, table sugar is a simple carbohydrate. When foods that contain refined sugars are eaten, a variety of things happen in your body:

- Your body releases serotonin, a brain chemical that makes you feel calmer.

- Your blood adrenaline level might increase from two to ten times the level it was prior to a sugary snack as shown in a 1990 study at Yale. Some children were found to have the highest increase in adrenaline, which might explain why some kiddos get wild after eating sugar.

- You might feel a "high" similar to the effect you might get from alcohol and other drugs, due to an increased release of brain neurochemicals, such as dopamine, nor-epinephrine, and serotonin. You can become addicted to this "high"!

- You might become more focused upon tasks. Adding a touch of caffeine, you'll be calm, but alert.

- If you eat more than 10 percent of your total calories from sugar, your nutritional status will suffer because you are choosing empty calories versus calories from nutrient-dense foods.

- Eating sugary foods might cause your digestion to slow down. Because of this, some researchers believe food is not digested properly, allowing larger particles of food to enter your bloodstream, setting the stage for food allergies.

- Each time you eat refined sugars or carbohydrates, you'll lose some of the trace mineral chromium through your urine. Chromium is needed for proper sugar fat and protein metabolism.

- Eating too many sugars might cause swings in your mood and energy levels.

Sad State of Affairs: High-sugar diets have been scientifically linked to higher levels of tooth decay. Other conditions related to a high sugar diet are diabetes, hypoglycemia, constipation, arthritis, gallstones, yeast infections, obesity, cancer, heart disease, and osteoporosis, to name but a few!

Action Tips:

- Eat a well-balanced diet with plenty of complex carbohydrates, a moderate amount of protein, and low amounts of fat.

- Eat fresh fruit such as strawberries, blackberries, raspberries, and apples. These are all high in fiber, which will slow the release of sugar into your bloodstream, preventing a fast drop or "lull" in energy.

- Use sugar as a treat on a weekly basis, *not* on a daily or hourly basis.

- Eat a sugary food with other nutritious foods in order to buffer its impact upon your body.

- Brush your teeth after eating any sugary and/or starchy food.

FMI:

The GL Diet for Dummies, Nigel Denby and Sue Baic, John Wiley & Sons Ltd., West Sussex, England, 2006

Taking a stroll after a meal could help you digest your food up to 50 percent faster.

Go Green!

Rome was not built in a day.
—Proverb—

Did You Know: What's green, served hot or cold, and has been shown to enhance weight loss and prevent diseases such as cancer and lower blood lipids? Green tea, of course! It's making quite the stir in the West even though archaeologists speculate the people of both China and India have been using green tea for more than five thousand years! Health experts have known Westerners had a higher incidence of cancer, heart disease, diabetes, and obesity and were perplexed as to why those in the East were just plain healthier. Green tea, and its primary component, EGCG, has been identified as one of the primary elements responsible for keeping Easterners healthy.

The Chinese & French Connection: For quite sometime to researchers it was somewhat of a mystery as to why the French stayed so slim and had a lower risk of cardiovascular disease compared to those in the West. They identified the regular habit of imbibing on red wine as a primary key to living a long and healthy life as a Frenchman or woman. Scientists honed in on a very important component in red wine called reservatrol. Resveratrol is a member of the super powered antioxidant family of polyphenols, known for their ability to protect against damage from excesses in smoking and eating a high fat diet. It just so happens the skins of red grapes are high in polyphenolic compounds such as resveratrol. Green tea contains EGCG, resveratrol's counterpart. Yet, EGCG, known also as a "catechin" (pronounced kat-a-kin!) packs twice the antioxidant punch of resveratrol! For example, green tea drinkers, in Japan, show a very low incidence of heart disease, in spite of more than 75 percent of the population smokes.

A Plethora of Benefits: Used medicinally in China, Japan ,and Thailand, green tea is commonly used to treat a wide array of ailments. Japanese researchers at the Saitama Cancer Research Institute noted fewer recurrences of breast cancer, and the disease spread much more slowly in those women who drank five or more cups of green tea daily. Scientists at the University of Purdue concluded there is an element in green tea that prevents the growth of cancer cells. Prevention of rheumatoid arthritis is possible if you drink four or more cups per day, according to a team at Cleveland's Western

Reserve University. Plus, green tea drinking decreases the abnormal formation of blood clots. And since EGCG is such a potent antioxidant, it is able to protect cells from invasion of bacteria and other offenders, thus boosting the immune system and helping the body resist infection.

But Wait, There's More! Green tea destroys bacteria responsible for tooth decay. It also has a thermogenic effect on the body and has been shown to facilitate weight loss. A group of subjects who did not change what they ate or typically did for activity, experienced an increase in metabolic rate, by 4 percent, when given green tea extract. Green tea is thought to have a thermogenic effect upon the body, revving up the fat burning engine!

Fat Chance: A green tea drinker will experience less absorption of triglycerides and cholesterol, and excretion of fat from the body is increased. Some studies show a decrease in total blood fats, including LDLs, the bad cholesterol, by drinking eight or more cups of green tea per day. Green tea does contain caffeine, only about 30 milligrams or so per cup, depending upon how much tea you use and how long you steep it for. Drinking decaffeinated green tea or taking a decaf green tea supplement may provide the same benefits without the caffeine "buzz."

The Calm Component: Green tea, especially the decaffeinated kind, acts as a mild sedative. L-Theanine, an amino acid found in green tea, raises the levels of serotonin in various important parts of your brain. L-Theanine is believed to be a non-sedating relaxant that works primarily by stimulating the brain's production of alpha waves and calming amino acids such as dopamine, gamma-aminobutyric acid, and tryptophan. Alpha brain waves are associated with a state of relaxed alertness, and studies show that people who produce more alpha brain waves have less anxiety.

Green or Black? What's the difference between green and black tea? Green tea leaves are steamed. This process prevents the EGCG compound from being oxidized. Black and oolong tea leaves are made from fermented leaves, which convert the EGCG into other compounds. The fermentation process makes oolong and black teas much less effective in preventing and fighting various diseases.

How Much? While some companies that sell green tea state that ten cups per day are necessary to reap maximum health benefits, a University of California study on its cancer-preventative qualities concluded that you could probably get the desired level of polyphenols by drinking two cups per day.

Action Tips:

- Drink one to two cups of green tea a day.

- Don't like the taste? Try a decaf green tea supplement.

- Don't boil green tea. Heat water then let it rest for a few minutes. Add tea. Then steep. Boiling may change the flavor.

Relative to its size, the tongue is the strongest muscle in the human body.

Be a Healthy Cook

If you think you can, you can.
And if you think you can't, you're right!
—Mary Kay Ash—

Did You Know: One of the most powerful ways for you to impact your health is to learn to prepare foods keeping your life in mind. Eating a diet high in greasy fats and refined carbohydrates and low in valuable whole grains, and fresh fruits and vegetables is one way you can shorten the length of your life. You don't have to be a chef in order to learn how to make food that is both tasty and healthy! Here are a few hints to help you on your way:

- Have an abundance of whole grains, fresh vegetables and fruits, and plenty of fresh herbs on hand at all times.

- When sautéing, use a "seasoned" iron skillet. Wipe the skillet with a small amount of olive oil. Minimal fat is needed with this method.

- Never boil fresh or frozen vegetables. Use a steamer basket instead. Cook veggies just until tender. Do not overcook so that you'll retain optimal nutrient content.

- Use the leftover water from steaming vegetables in stews or vegetables soups to add an extra nutrition punch!

- To prevent the growth of harmful bacteria, always keep eggs, meat, chicken, cooked beans, and rice in a refrigerator that is kept cooler than forty-five degrees Fahrenheit. Throw away any cracked eggs. Always wash all surfaces including your hands after working with raw chicken or turkey.

- Substitute evaporated skimmed milk for cream in recipes that require it.

- Instead of using salt, try using herbs such as dill, basil, and rosemary or spices such as curry and cumin.

- Prepare your own salad dressing with extra-virgin olive oil, balsamic vinegar or lemon juice, and garlic.

- Prepare gravies, sauces, and soups ahead of time, and place them in the fridge. You might easily remove the layer of fat that has solidified on the surface.

- Place a paper towel on the surface of the hot soup. It will absorb the fat layer right off the top!

- Never deep fry. Try grilling, baking, roasting, and sauté-ing as healthy alternatives.

- Use "ghee" or clarified butter if you need to use some form of fat besides olive or canola oil. It's high in mono-unsaturates and tastes great.

- To perk up brown rice, sauté the grain in the bottom of the pan before you add the water. Add a touch of sea salt and onion for flavor.

- Use tamari instead of soy sauce—it's much lower in sodium.

- Use fresh fruit for desserts or healthy garnishes.

Ahead of Your Time? If cooking is a hassle, and you can't seem to fit it into your schedule, simply devote one after-noon to "pre-prepare" big batches of your main staples such as chicken, brown rice, beans, etc. Divide them up into the proper portions and freeze! Remove your choice of food from the freezer and place it in the fridge to safely thaw. Prepare a fresh green salad, a cooked vegetable, and a whole grain to complement the dish. Add a piece of whole fruit for dessert and you're set!

Women who take birth control pills and smoke one pack of cigarettes per day are twelve times more likely to have a heart attack.

Take Your Alcohol Lightly

Most folks are about as happy
as they make their minds up to be.

—Abraham Lincoln—

Did You Know: People who indulge in a glass of wine on a daily basis might live longer than those who drink too much or who don't drink at all! Light drinkers, or those who drink one drink per day such as 5 ounces of wine, 1.5 ounces of eighty proof, or a 12 ounce beer, have a slightly lower risk of stroke than those who abstain. On the other hand, heavy drinkers (three or more drinks per day) have a two and a half times greater risk of suffering from a stroke than nondrinkers. Before you stock up on your favorite spirits, be forewarned that your liver loathes more than two drinks per day. People who drink are also more likely to be in car accidents, develop certain types of cancer, and commit suicide.

The Nitty Gritty: Alcohol weighs in at 7 calories per gram. Your body metabolizes it as if it were sugar and a fat combined. You might use some of the calories for energy but would be more likely to store them as fat. Alcoholic beverages usually do not contain significant amounts of nutrients needed for optimal health. As a matter of fact, alcohol might even deplete your body of vitamins B1, B2, B6, and B12, all valuable nutrients for the health of your nervous system. Vitamin C, vitamin K, zinc, magnesium, and potassium might also be lost.

Toast to Good Health! When we lift our wine glasses and toast to a long and healthy life, we may also be holding in our hands the beverage to make that happen. Researchers have found a substance in red wine, called resveratrol (res-ver-a-trol), that may help you live longer! The skin of red grapes is the most abundant source of resveratrol, a unique antioxidant that red grapes produce in great amounts as a defense against fungi. In the winemaking process, fermentation produces the resveratrol, and it's then preserved when the wine is bottled—otherwise the substance would vanish in days. Scientists have suggested that resveratrol acts as an antioxidant, mopping up harmful free radicals that damage cells. Resveratrol is about twenty to fifty times as effective as vitamin C alone as an antioxidant. And it acts synergistically with vitamin C enhancing the effects of each. Resveratrol has an anti-clotting effect that prevents the formation of blood clots in the blood vessels. Plus it may have anti-cancer effects as well. Resveratrol may extend the lifespan by having the same effect upon the body as calorie restriction. Calorie restriction can activate an enzyme called SIR2, which is thought to extend lifespan by stabilizing your DNA. Resveratrol is a small molecule that mimics calorie restriction. When you drink a glass of red wine, your body thinks it's being deprived of food. When this happens, genes are switched "on" that repair DNA. The end result? Your "hungry" body may not be as adversely affected as it would be on a calorie-rich diet!

Beer: Can You Drink to Your Health? The next time you enjoy your favorite brew, you might be doing your heart, eyes, and brain a favor. Drinking beer in moderation may have significant health benefits. According to a study from the University of Texas Southwestern Medical Center, adults who drink one to two beers per day may have a 30 percent to 40 percent lower rate of coronary heart disease compared with nondrinkers. Beer is rich in the antioxidant chemicals known as phenols and has a similar amount that is contained in red wine. The antioxidants in alcoholic beverages may be responsible for alcohol's health benefits including protecting against heart disease, cancer, and some other diseases. The antioxidant contents of red wine and beer are the same.

The up and the Down: Alcohol has a split personality when it comes to health in general. Let's take a look at the up side:

- Studies have shown that people who have one drink per day have a heart disease risk 21 percent lower than non-drinkers.

- Those who imbibe are 22 percent less likely to die of a stroke—two drinks per day being the limit—the stroke risk increases if you go beyond!

- According to a study at the Kaiser Permanente Medical Center in Oakland, California, people who had one to two drinks per day had a lower risk of coronary artery disease than nondrinkers.

- The American Cancer Society found, in a twelve-year study involving a million Americans in twenty-five states, that moderate alcohol intake has an "apparent positive effect on coronary heart disease."

- Moderate drinkers have higher levels of the protective cholesterol HDL.

- Researchers have also found that alcohol eases the impact of the stress on your body.

- Finally, if you have one drink per day, you'll be less likely to have a heart attack or stroke caused by blood clotting, because alcohol in the blood makes the platelets less sticky.

Now, for the Downside:

- Some studies have found an increased risk of stroke in people who have more than two drinks a day.

- If you drink, you have a lower overall risk of dying of cancer, but you are more likely to die of cancer of the mouth, throat, and esophagus. If you are a heavy beer drinker—five or more beers a day—you double your risk of rectal cancer.

- In the Harvard University Nurses Health Study of eighty-seven thousand women, it was discovered that women who have one drink per day have an increased risk of breast cancer. The National Cancer Institute found a 20 percent greater risk of breast cancer in women if they had one to four drinks a day. Their risk went up by 89 percent at five drinks daily.

So, Who Shouldn't Drink?

- If you have a family history of alcoholism or other substance abuse problems, just say no!

- Women who are pregnant should not imbibe! Studies indicate your baby might be smaller if you drink. Excessive alcohol during pregnancy might cause heart defects, retardation, facial deformities, or low birth weight.

Reformed Alcoholics: If you go back to drinking, your chances of dying will be almost 20 percent greater than the rest of the population.

Action Tip: Evaluate your lifestyle. If you use alcohol in a healthy manner, don't worry about it; just keep all the facts in mind! If you have trouble going a few days without a drink, you might have a problem, especially if it runs in your family. If alcohol is a barrier in your personal relationships, you should seek help in a treatment program.

FMI:
Alcoholic Anonymous
A.A. World Services, Inc. P.O. Box 459,
New York, NY 10163
(212) 870-3400 web: www.aa.org

The average American eats sixteen pounds of pasta each year.
An Italian eats a whopping fifty-five pounds annually!

Clear the Air

*I am not afraid of storms for
I am learning how to sail my ship.*
—Louisa May Alcott—

Did You Know: Toxins in your personal space, such as in your home or office, might make you feel a little lightheaded, tired, or irritable. If you experience frequent headaches, upset stomachs, and runny nose allergies and can't really identify the cause, you might be reacting to "xenobiotics."

Xeno-What? Xenobiotics (pronounced zee-no-biotics) is simply a fancy name for foreign chemicals. If your diet is primarily made up of processed foods, the water you drink is plain old tap water, and the air you breathe is loaded with chemical contaminants, you are exposing yourself to a wide variety of "xenos." When too many of these "xenos" enter your body, and your diet-and-exercise program isn't up to snuff, your health might be less than optimal.

The "Xeno-Free Radical" Connection: Here's how it works: If you're continuously exposing yourself to all sorts of chemicals (such as paint fumes, pesticides, strong cleaning products, and other types of obvious pollutants); eating a diet high in refined foods and low in whole grains, fresh fruits, and vegetables; drinking regular tap water; and are under stress, then "Free-Radical Overload" might occur. This simply means that all the "xenos" or foreign chemicals that make contact with healthy cells might cause the formation of free radicals. These free radicals lead to destruction of healthy cells, possibly leading to a breakdown of a healthy immune system and, in extreme cases, cancer. Children are especially sensitive to "xenos," because they metabolize things so rapidly.

"Xeno" Alternatives? If you're tired of being sick and tired, you might want to clean up your home and office environments. You never know what might happen. Check out these alternatives.

- Open your drains with a natural drain cleaner. Pour one-quarter cup of baking soda and one-half cup of white vinegar down your drain, wait a few minutes while the clog bubbles away, then rinse with hot water.

- For a natural furniture polish, mix two parts olive oil with one part lemon juice.

- To naturally clean your laundry, check out vegetable-based detergents.

- Leery of pesticides? Place dry bay leaves on your pantry shelves to deter roaches.

- Purchase bottled water or a water purification system for your home.

- Open windows frequently to allow circulation of fresh air. Sunshine helps to kill bacteria and molds in the air as well.

- Fill your home or office with plants. Green plants are natural air purifiers and also add valuable moisture and oxygen to your indoor environment! (A five-foot areca palm plant introduces two and a half cups of water to the air daily!) Ficus trees, ivies, and airplane plants are great natural air conditioners. Mold-sensitive individuals need to beware of an increased mold level that occurs as you add more plants to an internal environment. Using air filters such as an H. E. P. A. (High Efficiency Particulate Arresting) Filter for molds and an activated charcoal filter for chemicals will alleviate many of these concerns. Everyone would benefit from using one or both types of air filters in the home or office.

- If you live in a new home, be sure to ventilate well to allow the new products to "breathe."

- When you bring your dry cleaning home, remove the plastic bags and hang your clothes near an open, sunny window!

- Go the natural fiber route when it comes to what you wear and what you sleep on! Cotton, wool, and silk are wonderful natural fabrics typically free of chemical finishes that are normally found on synthetic fabrics. The chemical finishes found on polyester, acrylic, and nylon are made from petrochemicals, members of the "xeno" family. No-iron sheets have a finish made from formaldehyde, a pretty potent "xeno"!

- Instead of mothballs, use cedar chips or special wood treated with cedar oil.

Action Tip: Follow the recommended advice listed above. If you want to feel your best, clean up your act by eating better, exercising, learning to control stress, and as an added bonus, cut back on your exposure to "xenos."

FMI:
The American Environmental Health Foundation, 8345 Walnut Hill Lane, Suite 225, Dallas, Texas 75231
Phone: 214-361-9515 web: www.aehf.com

The Environmental Health Center—Dallas, 8345 Walnut Hill Lane, Suite 220, Dallas, Texas 75231 USA
Phone: 214.368.4132 web: www.ehcd.com

Fifteen percent of household dust is made up of human skin cells.

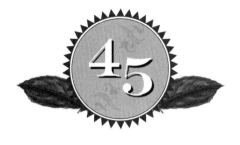

Maximize with Magnesium

Direct your eye inward and you'll find a thousand regions in your mind yet undiscovered.

—Henry David Thoreau—

Did You Know: Magnesium is of utmost importance as calcium's primary partner in your cellular dance. This magic mineral is called nature's tranquilizer because it is directly responsible for the relaxation action of your muscles. Magnesium is also known as nature's laxative! Alongside calcium, magnesium helps to keep your bones and teeth strong, your blood pressure down, and your metabolism rolling. Fifty percent of the magnesium in your body is found in the skeleton, 45 percent as chief components of fluid balance within your cell membranes, and the remaining 5 percent are found in your tissues. Magnesium is a vital cofactor in more than 300 different enzymes in the body. It is required for digestion, transmission of nerve impulses, cardiac electrical conduction, muscle function, antioxidant enzyme activity, hormonal balance, and maintaining life-sustaining ratios of electrolytes within cells. The ability of magnesium to help dissolve abnormal deposits of calcium is one of the most profoundly anti-aging effects of any mineral. The RDA for magnesium is 400 milligrams, but the average American diet only supplies between 200 and 350 milligrams per day.

Magical Magnesium: Magnesium might very well be one of the most important minerals in your body. Here's more info:

- Dr. Corey Slovis of Vanderbilt University Medical Center found that most patients who have suffered myocardial infarctions or heart attacks were deficient in magnesium. After giving magnesium though IVs, Dr. Slovis and other physicians found a significant drop in the death rate that usually occurs within thirty days of the first attack. That's a drop of 12 to 25 percent in mortality!

- People with high blood pressure at the University of Southern California were given a diet rich in magnesium and experienced a significant drop in blood pressure levels!

- Taking magnesium with calcium at bedtime helped induce relaxation in subjects who had trouble sleeping.

- A study of psychiatric patients found that those who were markedly deficient in magnesium were agitated, depressed, and sometimes hallucinated. Why? Anti-psychotic drugs deplete magnesium!

- Low magnesium levels might aggravate blood sugar problems such as diabetes.

- Women with PMS symptoms tend to have low magnesium levels in their bloodstream. A connection?

Bump Up the Mag! Whole grain cereals have about 10 percent of the RDA of magnesium. Other rich sources include figs, almonds, nuts, seeds, dark-green leafy vegetables, lemons, grapefruit, black strap molasses, wheat germ, soybeans, oatmeal, and brown rice. When cooking vegetables, be sure to steam or boil in a small amount of water, as magnesium is lost pretty quickly. Also, cook for the minimal amount of time possible.

Action Tips:

- Be aware of your mineral balance and eat a wide variety of foods including plenty of unrefined, whole grains, dark-green leafy vegetables, and other foods listed above.

- If you have trouble sleeping through the night, you might be deficient in magnesium. Take a calcium-magnesium supplement one hour before you go to bed.

- In a magnesium supplement, look for organic forms of magnesium such as magnesium citrate, magnesium succinate, magnesium aspartate, magnesium lactate, and magnesium taurinate are well-absorbed forms. Magnesium chloride is a well-absorbed inorganic form.

People who hate the taste of cabbage might not be able to metabolize certain chemicals in the leafy food, due to a gene passed on from Mom and Dad!

Keep Protein in Perspective

One cannot think well, love well, sleep well,
if one has not dined well.

—Virginia Woolf—

Did You Know: Protein is one of the major nutrient components of a well-balanced diet. Your body needs to acquire a specific amount of protein on a regular basis in order to literally maintain the integrity of almost every single cell in your body, including your bones, hair, teeth, nails, skin, etc. Your skeletal muscles, like your biceps, are chiefly comprised of protein tissue. Your brain, liver, kidneys, and even your heart are all heavily reliant upon protein for the rebuilding of their cells that have naturally died off. Collagen, the connective tissue that literally holds your body together, is also pure protein. Protein not only helps rebuild tissues and collagen, it also is necessary for regulating the fluid or water balance in your body. Protein-based cells make it possible to transport nutrients and oxygen through your bloodstream and into and out of cells. Antibodies, your immune system's "soldiers," are also protein-based. Protein is truly one of your body's major players in the physiological game!

The Essentials: Proteins are actually made up of smaller protein chains. These chains are called peptides and are made of smaller components called amino acids. There are eight essential amino acids that we must obtain through our diet. The amino acids are the true building blocks of your entire system. Your liver manufactures approximately 80 percent of the amino acids that your body needs, and your diet supplies the remaining 20 percent needed in the form of essentials.

If It Works for the Marines: Protein is needed after exercise especially since during intense exercise your muscle fibers are broken down and in need of repair. Protein is essential to repair damaged fibers. Researcher performed a study with Marine recruits that showed some amazing results. In boot camp, recruits from six platoons were assigned to one of three treatment protocols during fifty-four days of basic training. Each day after exercise, one group of Marines received a placebo drink containing zero calories; another received a control drink containing 8 grams of carbohydrate and 3 grams of fat; and the last group received a drink containing 8 grams of carbohydrate, 10 grams of protein, and 3 grams of fat. Compared to placebo and control groups, the protein-supplemented group had an average of 33 percent fewer total medical visits, 28 percent fewer visits due to bacterial/viral infections, 37 percent fewer visits due to muscle/joint problems, and 83 percent fewer visits due to heat exhaustion.

How Much Is Enough? Unfortunately, until recently, the dietary guidelines presented by the United States Department of Agriculture (USDA) were strongly influenced by the meat and dairy industry. It wasn't until recently that nutritionists and biochemists associated directly with the USDA began to take a serious look at the previous dietary recommendation and realized that health problems might be associated with excessive protein intake. Most protein sources that were typically being recommended were also high in saturated fat, known now to be the primary cause of elevated cholesterol levels.

A Closer Look: When you eat protein, which is essentially 4 calories per gram, your body will break it down in the digestive tract into the individual amino acids. These separated amino acids are then transported into your bloodstream where they come together to form other proteins designed for specific metabolic purposes.

Too Much for Some: High-protein diets are generally well tolerated by healthy adults. But a dramatic increase in protein-rich foods may be dangerous for people with liver or kidney disease. They lack the ability to rid their bodies of waste products from the metabolism of proteins. Although high-protein diets generally aren't harmful for people in good health, they may increase the risk of kidney stones and osteoporosis. A diet that is high in protein may also limit disease-fighting foods, such as fruits, vegetables, and whole grains. In addition, many high-protein foods—such as meat, milk, and eggs—are high in fat and cholesterol. So choose your sources of protein wisely. Good choices include fish, beans, and lentils, which are lower in fat and cholesterol, and low-fat dairy products. If you have kidney or liver disease or any chronic health condition, talk to your doctor before starting a new diet.

Nitrogen News: Protein is the only nutrient you eat that is primarily made up of nitrogen. The primary by-product of nitrogen being metabolized is urea or uric acid. Urea is toxic to your tissues, therefore, your body wants to move it on out as quickly as possible. Urea moves from your liver to your kidneys. Your kidneys then begin to work very hard to flush the urea out of your system, via the urine. When your diet is out of balance, containing way too much protein, your kidneys enlarge a bit, causing some pressure that might damage some of the tubules where blood filtration takes place. As we age, we typically lose a small amount of our kidney function, with elderly adults only using about 80 percent of their original kidney power. If a person has a defect in their kidneys obtained through their parents' genes or through a physical accident, researchers have found that a high-protein diet could be detrimental to the person's health.

Calcium Takes a Ride: In addition to general kidney problems, calcium depletion is another problem found when a body is working very hard to get rid of urea. The urine that leaves carrying urea also takes calcium out for the ride. Your body needs calcium for a wide variety of biochemical activities. If calcium is leaving your body and you are not getting more high-quality calcium through what you eat, your bones and teeth become self-sacrificing! Some feel too much protein might be directly linked with osteoporosis. Other researchers such as Dr. Willard Visek of the University of Illinois Medical School believe another by-product of protein digestion, nitrogen-based ammonia, might be a major cause of cancer of the colon. He has found that the more ammonia found, the higher the incidence of cancer.

Whey to Go! When choosing proteins, you should look for high quality proteins. Whey enhances glutathione production, one of your body's most powerful antioxidants, which boosts immunity. Whey protein supplements show high levels of protein bioavailability and are rapidly digested. Whey protein offers several other health benefits like stronger bones, weight loss, and just plain overall a better sense of well being. Whey protein is also sometimes used to help speed the healing of wounds or burns.

Hooray for the USDA! With the recent release of the new food pyramid guidelines, protein recommendations have become much more specific. The USDA is now recommending two servings per day, each no bigger than a deck of cards, or approximately 5.5 ounces total per day. It's really going to take some adjustment for the typical American who normally eats two to three times that amount daily! Pregnant women need 30 extra grams each day, and breast-feeding moms should add 20 grams. Simply multiply .36 by your present body weight and the number you obtain is the amount of protein grams you require daily. Endurance athletes (marathon runners, long distance swimmers, cyclists, and triathletes) need approximately 60 percent more protein than the average person, and bodybuilders should increase their amount by about 12 percent.

Get Your Protein Here! Lean, white meat chicken or turkey, flank steak, buffalo, wild game, cold-water fish, and eggs are all excellent sources of complete protein. Most vegetables, fruits, and carbohydrates contain small to large amounts of protein. Balance is the key in order to obtain the right "mix" of vegetable proteins. (See "Be A Semi-Vegetarian.")

Action Tips:

- Calculate your own protein requirement. It should approximate 10 percent to 15 percent of your total daily calories unless you fall into one of the extra protein categories as listed above.

- Divide your protein throughout each of your meals. Be sure to always have some form of complex carbohydrate along for the ride so that your protein will be specifically used for rebuilding your body and not burned as calories because of an energy deficit!

- Focus on lean sources of protein. If you want to cut the cholesterol and fat out of your breakfast, eat only the egg whites without the yolk. Try to eat beef no more than once a week. Eat more fish, lean chicken, and vegetarian sources.

FMI:
The USDA Food Pyramid Guidelines
Go to the Web: www.mypyramid.gov
for an interactive diet and nutrition platform.

Eighty-seven percent of Americans don't know
their cholesterol level.

The nicest thing about the future is that it comes one day at a time.

—Anonymous—

Put More Punch in Your Lunch

Did You Know: There is a new theory about why the French are healthier than Americans and most other Mediterranean cultures (besides the fact they drink more wine). It's because they eat their largest meal at lunchtime and snack less! Curtis Ellison, MD, of the Boston University School of Medicine, compared fifty Parisians with fifty Bostonians. He found that the French eat 57 percent of their total daily calories before 2:00 p.m.! After 2:00 p.m., they are unlikely to eat again until 7:00 or 7:30 p.m., when they usually consume lighter foods than they do at lunch.

The American Way: Americans that took part in the study were found to eat only 38 percent of their total daily calories before 2:00 p.m. and then they snacked three hours later. Americans typically have 2.9 snacks per day, usually making up to 22 percent of their total daily calories! The French only consume 1.1 snacks per day on average, making up only 7 percent of their total daily calories.

Better to Go Hungry? Some longevity specialists believe a low-calorie diet slows down aging. The theory maintains that if you are "working" without food, your body probably will produce less of the bad cholesterol or LDLs (the kind that create blockages in your arteries)

Action Tips:

- Eat a high-carbohydrate, low-fat breakfast. Lunch should be composed of four to six ounces of lean fish, a large salad, and two hefty servings of grains or "whole" carbo-hydrates.

- Drink room-temperature water with lemon! There's no fat to speak of and an added benefit will be heightened and alertness after lunch.

- Snack only on fresh whole fruit, water with lemon or lime, and some form of whole-grain carbs.

Chocolate contains a chemical also found elevated in the brains of people in love!

Your Brain: Use It or Lose It

Our nature consists in motion; complete rest is death.
—Blaise Pascal—

Did You Know: If you're over thirty, it is speculated that you'll lose 6 to 8 percent of your memory capacity every decade! Your brain's fate is dictated by a variety of factors, including what is genetically passed on to you by your biological parents. However, people who eat an optimal diet; exercise on a regular basis (especially those who participate in activities that require complex motor skills such as tennis or soccer); have a positive attitude; are social; and utilize visual memory techniques are much more likely to maintain optimal memory capacity not typical of the normal "aging" individual.

It Goes Slowly: Generally, different types of memory phase out at different times. "Semantic" memory, or the remembrance of general knowledge of the world and vocabulary, sticks around the longest, with first signs of loss typically not appearing until you're in your seventies. After the age of thirty-five, you might not remember names as well as you used to. "Spatial visualization" begins to go in your twenties, making it more difficult for you to recognize faces you've only seen on occasion. You'll also be more likely to forget where you parked your car in the mall parking lot! Different parts of your brain become less active, while others show more activity as you grow older. Physically, your brain begins to shrink as you age, and after you turn fifty, the loss of brain and nerve cells escalates. Harvard neurologist Dr. Marsel Mesulam theorizes that the loss of certain neurons or nerve cells in the brain and the activation of other locations is sort of an internal brain shift designed for fine tuning. As other cells die off, special brain cells containing a specific enzyme become more abundant in adulthood, which allows higher parts of your brain to become activated. Dr. Mesulam believes that this might be a result of developing "wisdom" in old age.

The Nuns Have "It": David Snowdon's fifteen-year old "Nun Study" at the Sanders-Brown Center on Aging at the University of Kentucky Medical Center has drawn national attention. Snowdon's book, *Aging with Grace: What the Nun Study Teaches Us about Leading Longer, Healthier and More Meaningful Lives,* reported that being mentally and physically active could stave off dementia. So what is the nuns' key to mental longevity? Like many nuns in the study, they don't believe in retiring! They found other occupations that keep their minds active. Other key components of the nuns' lifestyle are exercising regularly and remaining mentally active, i.e., reading, puzzles.

The Brain Drain: Smoking, air pollution, and a diet high in processed foods all contribute to brain cell or neuron depletion. Toxins or free radicals are introduced into your brain; these toxins cause nerve cells to oxidize and die off. Lack of aerobic exercise, stress, depression, minimal mental and social stimulation, and a deficiency of certain nutrients might also lessen your thinking ability and neurological integrity. So what's a person to do?

A "Memorable" Solution: Your brain needs plenty of blood flow, which can be provided through regular aerobic activity. If your cardiovascular system is healthy, more blood will travel to your brain, bringing along with it plenty of oxygen, vitamins, minerals, and glucose. Feeding your brain cells via increased blood flow from activity along with obtaining a nutrient-rich diet can result in more efficient brain functioning. Dr. Bill Greenough of the department of psychiatry at the University of Utah believes that aerobic activity that involves a certain amount of skill, tactical thinking, and visual alertness, such as in racquetball, tennis, or soccer, actually helps reverse the mental effects of aging! These types of activities force your brain to work overtime, which stimulates increased communication among nerve cells. The demand becomes so great that new cells and blood vessels are created in order to accommodate increased brain activity. Dr. Greenough has experimented with rats, forcing them to perform more complicated activities than their wheel-turning buddies, and found their brains became more developed! In addition, regular exercise helps people to be more able to deal with stress. There is a distinct connection between stress and mental shutdown. The more stressed-out you are, the more likely you'll be an absent-minded professor.

Other Brain Stuff: Being social and engaging in regular conversations with friends and associates stimulates your brain. Engaging in a variety of mental gymnastics such as playing games that demand the use of memory, being creative with art or writing, or solving crossword or other types of puzzles can get your brain rolling and keep it going! If you're depressed, as often occurs in old age, memory seems to go more quickly. The good news is, once the depression is identified and treated, memory often returns. Eating foods that are rich in antioxidants, such as beta-carotene, helps prevent destruction of brain cells normally caused by free radicals. Therefore, an optimal nutrient-rich diet is definitely in order for a healthy brain!

A More Serious Issue: In cases of Alzheimer's disease, there is a severe loss of mental functioning particularly pertaining to memory. The disease is passed on through a gene that turns into protein, whose sole function is to take cholesterol in and out of tissues and cells. This revolutionary new theory by Duke University Professor Allen D. Roses suggests that people with this gene might experience an abnormal buildup of plaque in the brain, hindering proper memory functioning. If the theory proves correct, a drug will be developed to hopefully arrest the genetic culprit.

Action Tips:

- Stay active aerobically—take up tennis!

- Be social. Read and discuss what you've read with friends.

- If your memory isn't what it used to be, if you feel lethargic, and if you lack an appetite and motivation, you might be depressed. Get treatment from a professional and chances are your memory will improve!

- Eat a diet rich in vitamins A, C, E, B, and selenium. Obtain them by consuming a variety of foods such as whole grains, fresh fruits and vegetables, cold-water fish, lean, skinless chicken, and plenty of water.

- Practice relaxation techniques, such as yoga, meditation, and listening to relaxing music.

Munch on one to two tablespoons of unsalted almonds daily five times a week and you'll lower your risk of heart attack by 50 percent!

It's Java Time!

When I look into the future, it's so bright it burns my eyes.
—Oprah Winfrey—

Did you know: A good old cup of java can lower your risk of diabetes, Parkinson's disease, liver disease, and cancer; lift your mood; treat headaches; and lower your risk of cavities. Once thought to be the "not so good" for you beverage, it turns out to be rather extraordinary. If you had to pick the leading source of antioxidants, what would you pick? Fruits? Vegetables? According Dr. Joe A. Vinson, a chemistry professor at the University of Scranton in Pennsylvania, Americans consume more antioxidants from coffee than any other food source. His study reported that the average adult consumes 1,299 milligrams of antioxidants daily from a cup of "Joe." Second closest competitor was tea at 294 milligrams, followed by bananas, 76 milligrams; dry beans, 72 milligrams; and corn, 48 milligrams. It seems that coffee does have some potential health benefits.

A Little Coffee History: Coffee can be traced to the highlands of Ethiopia in the ninth century. Then it made its way to Egypt and Yemen and by the fifteenth century, to Persia, Turkey, and Northern Africa. The beans were not allowed to leave certain countries so the Dutch ended up smuggling some out and began to grow it in Java, an island of Indonesia, which was the core of the Dutch East Indies. Exportation of the beans became commonplace. Eighteenth century men of culture loved coffee so much that that it was called an intellectual beverage. Coffee aroused interest not only as a refreshing infusion, but also for its healing powers; so that in a leaflet, printed in Milan in 1801, high credit was given by some physicians to coffee as a cure-all. After the war of 1812 in the United States, coffee became more popular due to tea importing restrictions.

A Good Habit! Coffee contains *hundreds* of biologically available compounds with only 2 percent of the total composition being caffeine. Coffee berries, or "beans" as they are commonly referred to, also contain trigonelline, amino acids, proteins, enzymes, carbohydrates, polysaccharides, antioxidants, oils, and at least 180 other compounds. One of the most abundant in coffee is chlorogenic acid, an antioxidant and an inhibitor of tumor formation. According to recent studies, moderate coffee drinking may lower the risk of colon cancer by about

25 percent, gallstones by 45 percent, cirrhosis of the liver by 80 percent, and Parkinson's disease by 50 percent to as much as 80 percent. Other benefits include 25 percent reduction in onset of attacks among asthma sufferers and, at least among a large group of female nurses tracked over many years, fewer suicides. In addition, some studies have indicated that coffee contains four times the amount of cancer-fighting antioxidants as green tea. Ironic, as over the past few years, coffee was thought to be a bad guy by the medical profession, linking coffee consumption as a major contributor to high blood pressure, heart disease, high cholesterol, high triglycerides, etc. It turns out those who drink coffee on a regular basis reap more health benefits over those who have an occasional cup. Nonhabitual coffee drinkers can have increases in heart rate, blood pressure, and blood sugar when they drink a cup of "Joe." Regular coffee drinkers don't have dramatic elevations in any of the three.

The "Wake Me Up" Cup: Many people can't start the day without their morning caffeine hit. Caffeine is one of the most widely consumed drugs in the world, with an average intake in the western world of 300 milligrams per day or the equivalent that is contained in two cups of coffee. Caffeine is a well-documented adenosine antagonist. Adenosine is responsible for feeling sleepy and a desire to sleep. Caffeine blocks adenosine from binding to its receptor or the "sleep trigger" and that is how it keeps you awake. Adenosine has begun to intrigue more and more sleep investigators. Many studies in animals have shown that blocking adenosine's actions in the brain increases alertness, while injections of adenosine or similar compounds induce apparently normal sleep.

So what makes cats sleep all day long? When cats are kept from napping by playing with them, levels of adenosine, build up in their brains and it is prevented from connecting with receptors that trigger sleep. The longer they stay awake, the higher the levels of adenosine. After they go to sleep, levels progressively drop off. What's true for cats is likely to be true for humans.

Dr. Feel Good: The brains of most coffee drinkers experience an increase in the release of dopamine, a neurohormone that is commonly associated with the pleasure system of the brain. When dopamine is elevated, dopamine elicits feelings of enjoyment and reinforcement to motivate a person to perform certain activities once previously experienced. Dopamine is released by naturally rewarding experiences such as by eating food, romantic activities, and even with drinking coffee. As a matter of fact, women who drink coffee have been shown to have higher libidos than those who don't. It is interesting to note, cocaine and amphetamines increase dopamine levels in the brain. Some researchers believe dopamine is released beforehand, just by anticipation. It's no wonder Starbucks® Coffee locations have become so popular!

The Fat Burner: In a 2006 study in BioMed Central Complementary and Alternative Medicine, green coffee beans were found to promote weight loss. The discovery mirrors earlier research on green tea, which was found to slightly increase metabolism and to speed up the body's ability to burn fat. Green coffee beans appear to have a more potent effect. The lead author of the study Hiroshi Shimoda reported, "If a human consumes one kilogram per day of food (2.2 pounds) containing 10 grams (.35 ounce) of green coffee bean extract for 14 days, the increase in body weight may be suppressed by 35 percent." Caffeine increases fat lipolysis or break down that increases free fatty acid utilization. Free fatty acids are an important source of fuel for many tissues since they can yield large quantities of energy.

Coffee and Diabetes: In the journal of *Diabetes Care,* a 2005 study reported that in a cross sectional study of 2,112 healthy women surveyed, coffee but not tea was associated with a significantly lower rates of type 2 diabetes. Coffee (both regular and decaffeinated) has lots of antioxidants like chlorogenic acid (one of the compounds responsible for the coffee flavor) and magnesium. These ingredients can actually improve sensitivity to insulin and may contribute to lowering risk of type 2 diabetes. Additionally, coffee was found to reduce the chances of developing cirrhosis of the liver: the consumption of 1 cup a day was found to reduce the chances by 20 percent, and 4 cups a day reduced the chances by 80 percent. So drink up.

Don't Get Carried Away: Caffeine, coffee's main ingredient is a mild addictive stimulant. And coffee does have modest cardiovascular effects such as increased heart rate, increased blood pressure, and occasional irregular heartbeat that should be considered. But, the negative effects of coffee tend to emerge in excessive drinking so it is best to avoid heavy consumption.

Action Tips:

- Invest in a good coffee pot.

- If possible, grind your coffee beans fresh, so you get optimum antioxidant benefits. The flavor will be better, too!

- Make smart choices of what you add to your coffee. Choose nonfat or low-fat steamed milk for your latte. Try a natural sweetener such as Stevia.

- Find a local StarBucks® and become a regular!

An average human drinks about 16,000 gallons of water in a lifetime.

Get Your Omega-3s

Virtue consists, not in abstaining from vice,
but in not desiring it.
—George Bernard Shaw—

Did You Know: There have been more than seven thousand reports, including nine hundred clinical trials on the study of fish oils and omega-3 fatty acids. Why? Because this essential fatty acid has been linked to all sorts of fantastic benefits including the improved health of the cardiovascular, nervous and hormonal release systems. It all started with the Eskimos of Greenland.

A Whale of a Tale: Greenland Eskimos, who eat large amounts of fat, have a low rate of heart disease. More than thirty years ago, Danish researchers speculated that a lower rate of heart disease in the Eskimos was linked to their diet primarily consisting of whale, seal, and fish. They concluded that their diet of whale, seal, and fish was rich in a type of fat that made the heart healthy difference. All eyes turned to omega-3s and how they can enhance overall health.

The Short List: Here are a few ways omega-3 fatty acids keep our bodies healthy:

* Reduces inflammation throughout your body

* Keeps your blood from becoming sticky

* Maintains the fluidity of your cell membranes

* Lowers the amount of lipids (fats such as cholesterol and triglycerides) circulating in the bloodstream

* Decreases platelet aggregation, preventing excessive blood clotting

* Increases the activity of a chemical called nitric oxide, which causes arteries to relax and dilate.

* Reduces the production of messenger chemicals called cytokines, which are involved in the inflammatory response associated with atherosclerosis

* Reduces the risk of becoming obese and improves the body's ability to respond to insulin by stimulating the secretion of leptin, a hormone that helps regulate food intake, body weight, and metabolism and is expressed primarily by adipocytes (fat cells)

* Helps prevent cancer cell growth

Omega-3s and Defibrillators? Fish oils in fatty fish like salmon might be even better than heart devices called defibrillators at preventing sudden death from heart problems. A recent study in the *American Journal of Preventive Medicine's* reported consuming fish oils ranked superior to defibrillators for saving lives. Using a computer-generated model, which raised omega-3 fatty acids from fish oils, would have about eight times the impact of distributing automated external defibrillators (AEDs) for saving patients with heart disease. AEDs are used to shock the heart back into action if it develops a fatal rhythm problem that can result in sudden death. The computer model analysis revealed that sudden death risk dropped 6.4 percent with adequate omega-3 fatty acid intake, while less than 1 percent death risk with access to AEDS.

Omegas Back in the Balance: Both omega-6 and omega-3 fats are essential for health. Hence, the term essential fatty acids. The key is to make sure their ratio to each other is balanced in our diet. Our bodies are designed to thrive on three to five times more omega-6 fatty acids versus omega-3s and not more. A Western diet is usually out of balance with eleven to thirty times more omega-6 than omega-3s! Why? In the '70s and '80s, many new foods were introduced containing polyunsaturated oils deemed heart healthy! Highly processed convenience foods became a hit too, normally rich in polyunsaturates. When in reality, it turned our fatty acid balance upside down! Many researchers believe the rising rate of inflammatory disorders in the United States is directly related to excessive omega-6s! Polyunsaturated corn oil, for example, is extremely high in omega-6s as compared to omega-3, ranking in at 46 to 1. Omega 6s in excess can cause inflammatory problems (See "Be a Little More Italian") and more. A healthier balance can be had if you choose your oils wisely! Canola oil ranks 2:1 ratio of omega-6 to omega-3. Soybean oil is 7:1; olive oil is 13:1; and flax oil is 1:3.

A Fishy Solution for Rheumatoid Arthritis: Fish oils can alleviate pain and inflammation in those with rheumatoid arthritis. Patients with the disorder were given fish oils and within three months were able to significantly cut back on their nonsteroidal anti-inflammatory drugs. Several test tube studies of cartilage-containing cells have found that omega-3 fatty acids decrease inflammation and reduce the activity of enzymes that destroy cartilage. Similarly, New Zealand green lipped mussel (Perna canaliculus), another potential source of omega-3 fatty acids, has been shown to reduce joint stiffness and pain, increase grip strength, and enhance walking pace in a small group of people with osteoarthritis.

Omega-3 Fatty Acids and Cancer: Eskimo populations in Alaska and some Japanese populations in northern Japan who consume diets based almost exclusively on fish seem to have a very low incidence of cancer, which increases with the westernization of their diet. Supplementing the diet of tumor-bearing mice or rats with oils containing omega-3 fatty acids has slowed the growth of various types of cancers, including lung, colon, mammary, and prostate. The omega-3 fatty acids have also been shown to increase the efficacy of various cancer chemotherapy drugs and of radiation therapy against cancer.

Too Much of a Good Thing? If you are taking omega-3 supplements, be sure not to take more than 3 grams per day. This is the amount the FDA states you should not exceed daily due to increased risk of various conditions such as increased bleeding, immune suppression, elevation of LDLs, and reduced glycemic control in diabetics. If you have been diagnosed with congestive heart failure, you should consult with your doctor before you take omega-3s. In some cases, the "beneficial" effects of omega-3s are not good for those who have less than optimal blood flow through the heart.

Action Tips:

- Eat fatty fish at least two times per week as recommended by the American Heart Association. Special note: One fish meal per week was associated with a 52 percent reduction in sudden cardiac death!

- Choose fatty fish like mackerel, lake trout, herring, sardines, albacore tuna, and salmon, which are high in two kinds of omega-3 fatty acids. You also want to look at the source of fish oils. Anchovies and sardines are lower on the food chain and so have less chance of incorporating mercury and other contaminants such as PCBs.

- Egg yolks, both chicken and duck, are a good source of omega-3 fatty acids.

- Omega-3 eggs found in the grocery store have 150 milligrams of omega-3s as compared to a regular egg measuring at only 18 milligrams. Plus, omega-3 eggs have six times more vitamin E than the more run-of-the-mill variety.

- If you go the supplement route, the FDA has approved up to 3 grams per day of fish oil (lower dose if oil is from fish liver!) safe for humans of all ages.

- Good plant-based sources of omega-3 fatty acids are:

  — Leafy green vegetables (spinach)

  — Nuts (walnuts, Brazil nuts, hazelnuts, pecans. Brilliant as a snack instead of sweets.

  — Seeds (especially sesame seeds). Choose a seeded roll when you go shopping.

  — Tahini—Tahini is a sesame seed paste that is used itself as a dip and also as a base for some Middle Eastern sauces such as curries, as a roux would be in European cooking.

  — Hummus—A great-tasting chickpea dip.

  — Oils—Soya bean oil, sunflower oil, canola oil, rapeseed oil, linseed/flaxseed oil. Most of these can be found in your local supermarket. Experiment when cooking, marinating, and dressing.

Your tongue print is as unique as your fingerprints!

Keep an Ion Your Health

No one knows what he is able to do until he tries.
—Pubilius Syrus (c.a. 50 B.C.)—

Did You Know: If you feel a sense of renewed energy after a clapping thunderstorm, or a sense of calm when you visit the seashore or sit by a waterfall, you are reacting to electrically charged particles in the air. Ions are invisible particles of the air, which, if they had all their parts, would be referred to as electrons. Ions are simply missing a piece of energy, which makes them either positively or negatively charged. Ions occur naturally in the air. You would find them, if you measured them, approximately one thousand to two thousand ions per cubic centimeter of air. The ratio of positive to negative (referred to as pos-ions and neg-ions), is 5:4. This is called an ion balance. If the balance goes out of whack, or the number of pos-ions increases dramatically, insects, animals, and most people can feel the difference and manifest their reaction in a variety of ways. Insects and animals become visibly more active and agitated when the pos-ions increase. People, on the other hand, might feel low energy or depression, suffer from insomnia, and have aggravated allergies, just to name a few symptoms.

Nature Gone Awry: The natural ion balance becomes imbalanced due to circumstances in nature, as well as a result of modern man's own doing. Man's concrete jungle causes the ion balance to become very distorted. In nature, an imbalance of ions can occur when a cool front in the atmosphere encounters a warm front. They sort of clash and create friction. When there are more positive ions, the charged air sometimes experiences a release of electricity such as when lightning is created during a thunderstorm. Lightning uses up much of pos-ions, leaving plenty of negative ions floating around. It is these negative ions that are associated with a sense of calmness in many people. Imagine your body being one big circuit of energy. The Chinese refer to this energy as "Chi." If you encounter negative ions, whose job it is to neutralize positive ions, your body's charge is neutralized. Negative ions are good; too many positive ions are detrimental to optimal physical and mental health.

The "Winds": At certain times of the year, there are certain places on the earth where an abundance of pos-ions are created, such as those called the Chinook winds along the Rockies or the Santa Ana winds in Southern California. Certain parts of Switzerland and many other places in the world are known to have these periodic winds that appear to make people highly agitated. Some get depressed and others complain of more illness during these times. (Remember all the reports of people shooting each other on the L.A. freeways? You've got it! It's usually during the Santa Ana winds.)

Who's the Lucky One? Researchers have found that 25 percent of all people are strongly affected by too many pos-ions, the next 50 percent are somewhat affected, with the remaining 25 percent appearing to be nonreactive.

Documents Please:

- There have been more than five thousand studies of the ion connection that have been documented worldwide. The conclusions are universal: Too many positive ions are detrimental to general well-being, and an abundance of negative ions is a good thing.

- When a group of people was studied in a situation where aggressive behavior was provoked, the conclusion was that people who leaned toward type-A aggressive behavior reacted with more hostility when the room was blasted with positive ions. Under the same provocation, with an abundance of negative ions, the subjects were much calmer and did not react aggressively.

- In both Russian and U.S. studies, plants grown under conditions with elevated positive ions experienced diseased and stunted growth.

- Forty male students were given the assignment to complete difficult computer tasks. When exposed to negative ions, their production was higher and they had fewer errors than when exposed to too many positive ions.

- In the June 1990 *Environmental Research Journal*, a study was reported where infectious microbes and bacteria were reduced by 40 percent to 50 percent in the air of a dental clinic with the use of negative ion generators—devices commonly used in other countries.

- In a Canadian study, as a measure of brain activity, listening tests were given to a group of seventy-three children. Their listening accuracy improved as more negative ions were introduced into the enclosed room.

- In Russia, researchers tried to raise small animals such as mice and rabbits in pure oxygen environments, without any ions at all. They all died within a few weeks. Conclusion? We need ions in order to properly assimilate oxygen molecules in our lungs!

- Burn patients at a Philadelphia hospital received negative ion "treatments" for fifteen minutes three times per day. In 75 percent of the patients, wounds healed at a faster than normal rate.

So, Now What? What is the deal at the seashore? It turns out that moving water creates negative ions. When saltwater pounds the beach or rocks, negative ions are being created! Fountains, creeks, rivers, and especially waterfalls, such as Niagara Falls, are fantastic negative ion generators. Maybe the honeymoon capital is really a result of humans seeking out the ultimate calming experience!

Action Tips:

- Figure out if you're one of those people who is sensitive to ion changes. If you are, you might want to make regular visits to a fountain or moving body of water. (The effects do last for a limited period of time after exposure.)

- Take showers, the ultimate negative ion generators.

- Open windows if you are in an enclosed building. Concrete buildings with lots of air conditioning and heating tend to build up pos-ion levels.

- Keep an open mind to possibilities of things that might affect your health even though you can't see them! And keep an "ion" your health!

FMI:
The Owners Manual for the Brain:
Everyday Applications from Mind Brain Research, Pierce J. Howard, PhD,
Bard Press, Austin, Texas, 2006

What percentage of men say they get to have too much sex?
One percent.

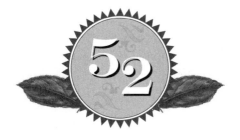

Jump Start Your Metabolism
with Herbs

Nothing can bring you peace but yourself.
—Ralph Waldo Emerson—

Did You Know: Globally, there are more than one billion overweight adults and at least 300 million of them are obese. Obesity poses a major risk for chronic diseases, including type 2 diabetes, cardiovascular disease, hypertension and stroke, and certain forms of cancer. Natural alternatives for weight loss may be the answer for many. Caffeine, capsaicin (the active ingredient in cayenne peppers), green tea, and other herbs may be used for weight loss and weight maintenance since they speed up the metabolic rate.

The "Weight" Game: You lose weight by burning more calories than you consume. If you can boost your metabolism, you will be able to burn more calories per day and lose weight, assuming you're following a healthy diet. Ever see some people who can eat all day long and not gain weight, such as teenagers? Due to increases in hormone production, their metabolism is revved up all day long, but as we all know that does not last for long. As you age, hormone levels shift, diets change, activity slows, and, thus, weight gain occurs for many people. You may be able to prevent this from happening by kick-starting your metabolism with herbs.

"Plant" It Out: Herbs are plant extracts that are being used to treat hundreds of ailments and conditions, including excess weight. Although they are only just gaining popularity in the West, they have long been a health maintenance staple in many other parts of the world. Don't think that herbs by themselves will cause weight loss. Herbs must be used in conjunction with your diet and exercise regimen in order to help you lose weight.

The Natural Solution: Herbs come in the form of supplements, teas, and even foods that will help you lose weight. There are several herbs that contain sympathomimetics that increase adrenaline. Xanthine compounds, found in coffees and teas, increase the body's basal metabolic rate to increase the burning of calories and fat, act as mild stimulants, and suppress the appetite. Herbs kick start the "thermogenesis," the process by which the body generates heat energy that burns fat. Those herbs reported to stimulate thermogenesis found in diet or metabolism formulas include the following:

Cinnamon—Cinnamon makes cells more responsive to the hormone insulin. Because insulin regulates glucose metabolism and controls the level of glucose in the blood, cinnamon may have the potential to delay or prevent adult-onset, or type 2, diabetes. A little bit of cinnamon added to your coffee or tea can make fat cells much more responsive to insulin and enhance weight loss.

Cayenne/Mustard—Cayenne pepper, actually a small red berry from the Capsicum annum plant, creates heat when taken into the body. (Capsaicin is the chemical that makes peppers hot.) One of the true natural stimulants for both energy and metabolism, it is believed that when cayenne pepper is used regularly it has anticancer properties, reduces pain and swelling, and is beneficial as a topical analgesic. It also stimulates circulation, aids in digestion, and breaks up congestion. Research suggests that cayenne increases the body's heat production and speeds up the metabolism of fats and carbohydrates. Cayenne may cause increased production of epinephrine and norepinephrine, which could account for the reduction in appetite. Scientists have found that people, who ate hot spicy foods, adding a teaspoon of red-pepper sauce and a teaspoon of mustard to their meals, raised their metabolic rates by as much as 25 percent. The hot spices also stimulate thirst, so you drink more liquids that also help in gaining less weight.

Black Pepper—Black pepper is derived from the pepper plant, a large woody vine that can grow to heights of more than thirty feet in the hot and humid climates of the tropics. Problems with digestion are increasing in frequency, and black pepper seems to be effective in improving the digestion, probably due to the way in which black pepper stimulates the taste buds. This stimulation of the taste buds notifies the stomach to increase its secretion of hydrochloric acid, improving the digestion of food once it reaches the stomach. Black pepper warms and relaxes muscles and dilates blood vessels to help remove toxins.

Ginger—Ginger has been recognized for its medicinal properties for thousands of years. It is the spice that is perhaps best known for its ability to help the digestive system. Ginger contains gingerols and shogoals, which are substances that may help to calm stomach acid and tone the muscles of the digestive tract. The thermoregulatory properties in ginger help regulate metabolism. Preliminary research, reported in the *International Journal of Obesity* in October 1992, shows that ginger boosts weight loss by calorie burning. By measuring a complicated series of reactions in rats, researchers found that ginger made the tissues use more energy.

Guarana—Guarana comes from the seeds of a South American shrub, most of which originated in Brazil. Traditional uses of guarana by natives of the Amazon rain forest include crushed seeds added to foods and beverages to increase alertness and reduce fatigue. The major active constituent in guarana is caffeine and similar alkaloids, such as theobromine and theophylline (which are also found in coffee and tea). Each of these compounds has well-known effects as nervous system stimulants. As such, they may also have some effect on increasing metabolic rate, suppressing appetite, and enhancing both physical and mental performance. Guarana also contains tannins, which act as astringents and may prevent diarrhea.

Coffee, the Amazing Elixir—For years, coffee was associated with having high blood pressure and being bad for the heart; however, these misconceptions are being refuted, and some advocates are even calling coffee healthy. (See "It's Java Time!") For instance, we know that regular consumption of coffee decreases the risk of type 2 diabetes. A recent study looked at energy expenditure and fat burning after caffeine or placebo ingestion, using placebo-controlled, double-blind conditions. Researchers studied ten older men, ages ranging from sixty-five to eighty, and ten younger men, ages nineteen to twenty-six, who were moderate consumers of caffeine. The metabolic rate or the rate they burned calories increased 11 percent in the younger men and 9.5 percent in the older group. Caffeine can also help dampen appetite; however, moderation is key.

Action Tips:

The most successful weight loss plans combine the following:

- Healthy eating

- Balanced nutrition

- Regular exercise, including cardio as well as resistance training

- Nutritional supplements

- Writing down all that you eat and drink in a food diary to prevent mindless eating!

- Adding one or two of the herbs in this chapter. Listen to your body.

- Never taking herbs in excess

A recent study indicates that those who take an annual vacation have less heart disease and a lower mortality rate.